The Secret Lemon Fix:

How Nature's #1 Disease-Fighting Fruit Can Radically Heal Your Body Every Day

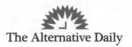

The Alternative Daily

This page intentionally left blank.

This page intentionally left blank.

Table of Contents

67 Ways to Use Lemons Every Day- Recipes for Health, Beauty and Home!

This page intentionally left blank.

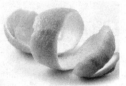

"We are living in a world today where lemonade is made from artificial flavors and furniture polish is made from real lemons."

—Alfred E. Newman

The Tart and Powerful Superfood

Lemons are one of the most affordable superfoods on the planet. For less than a dollar, you can help remedy and prevent an assortment of temporary and chronic ailments. Lemons are versatile fruits that can complement most dishes, so it's easy to sneak them into your diet.

The lemon is such a powerful fruit that many people are beginning to drink lemon water first thing in the morning to alkalize their bodies and get their morning vitamin C boost.

Others include lemons in comforting herbal teas, with raw honey to complement the healing properties in the tea blend.

You might be surprised to learn that there is enough information about lemons to make an informational book such as this. However, lemons deserve respect for their potent nutritional and medicinal properties—and don't forget that lemons are a great addition to your beauty and home cleaning regime, as well.

It's time for lemons to shine, and we have compiled the latest information on this little tropical wonder, with the added bonus of unique, cost-saving recipes for you to enjoy.

The Alternative Daily

Fascinating Facts about Lemons

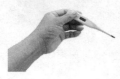

Lemons can prevent colds and flu

By boosting the immune system, the high quantity of vitamin C found in lemons helps your body fight off infection and viral ailments.

Lemons can help to break a fever

By increasing perspiration, lemons may help bring down a fever.

Lemons have been used to help treat cholera and malaria

Lemons can help your circulatory system. In fact, they have been used traditionally for centuries for their blood purification properties.

Lemons can stop a nosebleed

Lemons have antiseptic and anticoagulant properties, which means they can help disinfect an area and stop bleeding. When applied to the inside of your nostrils with a cotton ball, lemon juice may help to stop annoying nosebleeds.

Lemons can be used as a natural pain reliever

Lemons are naturally diuretic and may help relieve symptoms of rheumatism and arthritis by flushing out toxins and bacteria in your system.

Lemon juice can help to reduce gallstones

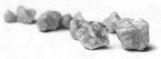

Drinking lemon water can help reduce gallstones and eliminate kidney stones by producing urinary citrate, which prevents the formation of crystals.

Lemons can help shrink your waistline

Lemons can aid in weight loss because they help speed up your metabolism. They may also help lower your risk of diabetes.

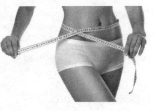

Lemon water can be used as a natural hairspray

Lemon water can be used as a hairspray replacement. It can also naturally lighten your hair. Best of all, lemon juice is actually beneficial to your hair and scalp! It reduces inflammation that causes dandruff and hair loss, and leaves your hair with a natural shine.

Lemon juice can reduce the pain of a burn

Apply lemon to the skin to help cool down a burn. It may even reduce the appearance of scarring from burn-related incidents. Lemon juice may also help reduce the pain associated with sunburns and bee stings.

Lemons can reduce the signs of aging

The antioxidants found in lemon help fight free radicals and reduce the signs of aging.

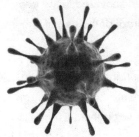

Lemons can help stop gum disease

Massaging your gums with lemon juice can help stop gum disease and eliminate the odor associated with it. Rubbing lemon juice onto a painful tooth may also help to eliminate the pain.

Lemons kill germs

Lemon is a great disinfectant because it kills germs and helps prevent the spread of bacteria. It can be used to clean floors, countertops, and tables.

Lemons repel insects

The scent of lemons is strong enough to repel mosquitos and other pests. Using lemon in your home, and especially in your kitchen, can help keep your surfaces safe from tiny invaders.

Read on for more amazing lemon facts, uses, and tips...

History of Lemons

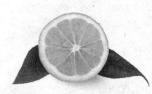

Lemons were developed as a hybrid of the lime and the citron. Although images depicting lemons have been found from Ancient Greece and Rome, historians believe that they were first cultivated in Ancient India 2,500 years ago on the hot, semi-arid Deccan Plateau.

The word "lemon" originates from the Persian word "limu," which is pronounced with a long "e" and a short "u." The first description of the lemon was discovered in the early tenth century treatise on farming by Qustus al-Rumi. Written proof of the use of lemons was first found in an early twelfth century Cantonese text.

Europeans were introduced to the lemon by the Arabs, who brought the fruit over to Spain in the eleventh century. Around that same time, lemons were also being introduced via trade to the African continent. The spread of lemons throughout Europe is attributed to the Crusaders, who found lemons growing in Palestine. Lemons appeared in the Azores in the late fourteenth century and were cultivated in Genoa, Italy in the fifteenth century.

Ibn Jami', personal physician to the ancient Muslim leader, Saladin, produced a treatise on the lemon. After the treatise was made public, the mention of lemons in literature grew throughout the Mediterranean region. As with several other fruits, the lemon was brought to the Americas by Christopher Columbus in his second voyage to the New World in 1493.

In the nineteenth century, lemons were highly prized by hard-working laborers, especially those working in coal mines. Lemons protected these workers from scurvy due to their abundance of vitamin C. In 1849, the demand for lemons was so incredibly high that producers charged the consumer one dollar per lemon, a price that would even be considered unreasonable by today's standards.

Florida has been a predominant producer of lemons in the United States since the sixteenth century. Today, the United States and Italy are considered two of the main producers of lemons in the world. Other major producers include Greece, Spain, Turkey, Israel, and Argentina.

Lemon Varieties

According to Sunkist, there are two main varieties of lemons that dominate the global marketplace: the Lisbon and the Eureka. Sunkist claims that these two varieties are so similar that many specialists can't tell the difference. The Lisbon and the Eureka are part of a group called "sour lemons," which are more tangy and acidic than the "sweet" varieties.

Other sour lemons include pink lemons and Ponderosa lemons. Pink lemons are popular for their use in pink lemonade, due to their slightly different flavor and beautiful rose color. The skin of this lemon is not pink, but green and yellow. It is the flesh within that is pink.

Pink lemons come from the variegated pink Eureka lemon tree. Ponderosa lemons come from the Ponderosa lemon tree. However, don't let the name fool you—Ponderosa lemons are actually not lemons at all. In fact, they are considered to be a lemon substitute. The juice of this yellow fruit is tart enough to be used as a replacement for squeezed lemon juice in recipes.

"Sweet lemon" varieties taste less sour and acidic when compared with most lemons on the market. Sweet lemons include Meyer lemons and Sanbokan lemons. Meyer lemons are not truly sweet, just milder than sour lemons. In other words, they don't make you pucker quite as much. They are heavier in weight and more juicy than typical sour varieties.

Meyer lemons are great for sweet dishes and for making lemon olive oil. Sanbokan lemons could be considered a lemon-orange hybrid. This type of lemon was first discovered in Japan in 1848. The Sanbokan resembles an orange with a prominent neck. As it matures, it even turns orange instead of yellow. It may look like an orange, but it tastes more like a lemon. Unfortunately, it is not considered marketable in the United States due to its orange color and excessive seediness.

There is also a lemon called the "rough lemon," which is a cross between an orange and a citron fruit. This fruit is often considered to be of low quality, so rough lemon trees are normally used as rootstock for other, more profitable lemon varieties.

Nutritional Information

According to the U.S. Food and Drug Administration, a medium lemon contains only 15 calories, is fat free, low in sodium, and has 5.4 grams of total carbohydrates, only 2 grams of which are sugar. Lemons are low-glycemic, alkalizing fruits that are loaded with a plethora of nutrients.

Lemons have dietary fiber to keep you regular, and contain a good amount of vitamin C. In fact, one lemon has 40 to 50 percent of your daily requirement for vitamin C! Lemons are also a good source of B vitamins, including thiamin, vitamins B2 and B6, riboflavin, and pantothenic acid. On top of that, they boast a wealth of minerals, including potassium, phosphorus, calcium, iron, manganese, magnesium, copper, and zinc.

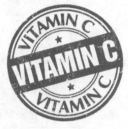

Lemon juice is commonly used in both savory and sweet dishes, drinks, and desserts. One fluid ounce of lemon juice contains only 7 calories. It contains 2.1 grams of total carbohydrates and only trace amounts of protein and fats. Although it has only 0.1 grams of both fiber and sugar, it still has a whopping 23 percent of your daily vitamin C needs!

Lemons are also rich in antioxidants, which give them their bright yellow color. These antioxidants help protect DNA from free radicals, eliminate toxins from the system, help prevent cancer, and may reduce the appearance of aging.

Nutrional Profile

Minerals in Lemons		Vitamins in Lemons
Potassium: 116 mg		Vitamin C: 44.5 mg
Calcium: 22 mg		Vitamin B1 (thiamine): 0.034 mg
Phosphorus: 13 mg		Vitamin B2 (riboflavin): 0.017 mg
Magnesium: 7 mg		Vitamin A: 18 IU
Sodium: 2 mg Iron: 0.5 mg Selenium: 0.3 mcg Manganese: 0.025 mg Copper: 0.031 mg Zinc: 0.05 mg		Niacin: 0.084 mg Folate: 9 mcg Pantothenic Acid: 0.16 mg Vitamin B6: 0.067 mg Vitamin E: 0.13 mg
Also contains small amounts of other minerals.		*Contains some other vitamins in small amounts.*

Scientific Research

From the first section of this book, you can see that lemons are widely regarded as cleansing agents that can detoxify your body, help prevent disease, and clean your surroundings. These seem like wonderful claims, but is there any evidence that suggests these seemingly outlandish health claims are true? Scientists have indeed put these claims to the test. The following are some of their results:

The Journal of Clinical Biochemistry and Nutrition published their findings on the effects of polyphenols within lemons on body weight. They put mice on one of three diets: a low-fat diet, a high-fat diet, and a high-fat diet that included lemon polyphenols. They found that lemon polyphenols actually suppressed not only body weight and fat deposits, but also obesity-related disorders such as insulin resistance, hyperlipidemia, and hyperglycemia.

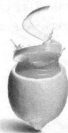

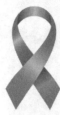 What about cancer? If we told you that lemons may help prevent and combat tumor cells, it may seem pretty far-fetched—but is it? A 2002 study published in the *Journal of Agricultural and Food Chemistry* revealed that the flavonoids in citrus fruits can actually help combat several forms of cancer, including melanoma, breast, colon, lung, and prostate cancers.

Another study, released by *Oxford Journals* in 1990, found that lemon oil can inhibit the inducement of cancer from carcinogens. Citrus pectin was also found to be effective against prostate cancer by actually slowing its progression, according to 2003 research released by *Prostate Cancer and Prostatic Diseases*.

What about other potentially deadly diseases? Research published in the 2010 edition of the *Journal of Basic and Applied Sciences* studied rabbits that were fed a high cholesterol diet for four weeks and were given lemon juice to determine the effect of lemons on hyperlipidemia.

As a quick reference, blood lipid content is a major determinant of developing heart disease. The results of the 2010 study showed that the lemon juice improved choles-terol, triglyceride, and lipoprotein levels, thus acting as a powerful protector against heart disease and stroke.

Lemon has been used for generations as a cleaning agent due to its antibacterial and antiseptic properties. A study published by *BMC Complementary and Alternative Medicine* in 2006 found that lemon oil is, in fact, antibacterial and was shown to be effective against multiple strains of bacteria.

The December 2008 edition of *Food Control* also published findings that demonstrate how lemons can be an effective antifungal agent, by showing how lemon oil can inhibit mold growth on food products. The researchers concluded that lemon oil and other citrus oils could replace chemical preservatives.

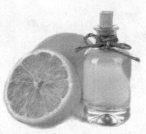

The Iranian Journal for Public Health published a study in 2003 on the use of lemon oil and lemon extract as mosquito repellents. Researchers found that lemon is in fact an adequate mosquito repellant, though not as potent as DEET. However, DEET has many potentially dangerous side effects, while lemon is natural and healthy. The researchers who performed this study also discovered that lemon oil is more effective than lemon extract at repelling mosquitoes.

There are also patents pertaining to the use of lemons in cosmetics, pharmaceuticals, and pet health products. These products use lemons for a variety of functions, including moisturizing, cleaning, treating hair and skin disorders in pets and humans, and fighting inflammation. There are even patents on health drinks that promote their lemon juice content as an anti-inflammatory agent. Researched published in 1997 by the *Journal of Agriculture and Food Chemistry* found that when gut bacteria comes in contact with lemon, the antioxidative effects remain active.

What Lemons Can Do for Your Health

Many of us love lemons for their fresh flavor and the pop they lend to so many recipes. However, lemons have a wide range of important health benefits, as well. Here are some to consider:

Anxiety relief

Since lemon contains a considerable amount of potassium, it may help to curb anxiety and depression. It has been found that low potassium levels in the body may contribute to both of these psychological disturbances, and the potassium boost that lemon provides may aid in bringing relief. Plus, the energy boost that you'll get from fresh lemon can help to elevate your mood in general.

Using lemon essential oil as aromatherapy may also bring about a lift in mood and potentially ease anxiety. It may help you to sleep better, as well. The authors of a 2008 study published in the journal *Tree and Forestry Science and Biotechnology* wrote:

"Traditional populations in several countries usually reference *Citrus* species as useful in reducing symptoms of anxiety or insomnia."

For an extra anxiety-relieving punch, try squeezing a wedge of fresh lemon into a cup of chamomile or lemon balm tea. To enjoy the aromatherapeutic benefits of lemon essential oil, try placing a few drops in a diffuser in your bedroom or study.

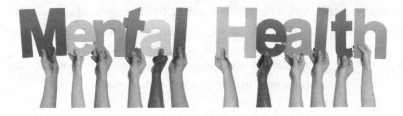

Blood pressure

The potassium found in lemon serves another important purpose: it may help to lower blood pressure. Potassium is an important mineral that helps to keep blood vessels soft and flexible. This, in turn, helps to reduce high blood pressure. Controlling high blood pressure levels may help to reduce the risk of heart disease and stroke.

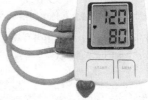

A 1998 study published in *Food Science and Technology International, Tokyo* tested the relationship between some of the components found in lemon juice on blood pressure in rats. On their experiment and its results, the study authors wrote:

"The effects of lemon juice and its crude flavonoids on blood pressure were examined using spontaneously hypertensive rats (SHR). The 5% diluted lemon juice was orally administered in the diet to SHR, and they tended to have a lower systolic blood pressure than the control rats after 90 days. The systolic blood pressure of SHR fed a diet containing crude flavonoids from the juice for 16 weeks was significantly lower than that of the control group…"

The vitamin B found in lemons is also beneficial to heart health.

Brain health

Although the peel of the lemon is frequently tossed in the garbage, it contains the phytonutrient tangeretin, which has been shown to have positive effects on brain disorders like Parkinson's Disease due to its neuroprotective qualities.

The effects of tangeretin on "rat models of Parkinson's disease" were examined by a 2001 study published in *NeuroReport.* The authors of the research wrote:

"These studies, for the first time, give evidence that tangeretin crosses the blood–brain barrier. The significant protection of striato-nigral integrity and functionality by tangeretin suggests its potential use as a neuroprotective agent."

So, instead of throwing out that peel, try adding lemon zest to your recipes. To avoid potential contact with dangerous pesticides, always choose organic lemons.

Cancer protector

Lemons contain 22 anti-cancer compounds. One of these is limonene—an oil that has been shown to halt the growth of cancerous tumors in animals.

A 2005 study published in the *Journal of Nutrition* found that the limonoids in citrus fruits protect cells from damage that can lead to cancer. Another study published in the *Journal of Agriculture and Food Chemistry* stated that limonoids can inhibit tumors in the mouth and stop the growth of cancer cells once a tumor has formed.

In addition, lemons also contain flavonol glycosides, which may help stop the division of cancerous cells.

On the cancer-combatting effects of flavonol glycosides and other citrus flavones, the authors of a 2001 study published in *Current Medical Chemistry* wrote:

"Citrus flavonoids encompass a diverse set of structures, including numerous flavanone and flavone O- and C-glycosides and methoxylated flavones. Each of these groups of compounds exhibits a number of in vitro and in vivo anti-inflammatory and anticancer actions."

The authors of another study, published in 2008 in the journal *Nutrition and Cancer*, explain:

"Dietary polyphenols are important potential chemopreventive natural agents. Other agents, such as citrus compounds, are also candidates for cancer chemopreventives. They act on multiple key elements in signal transduction pathways related to cellular proliferation, differentiation, apoptosis, inflammation, and obesity."

Canker sores

The antiviral and antibacterial properties of lemons can help to speed up the healing process when it comes to canker sores.

A 2004 study published in the *Journal of Pharmaceutical Sciences* found that an adhesive tablet which released citrus oil (along with other natural compounds, including magnesium salt) was more effective at treating canker sores than tablets without the infused compounds.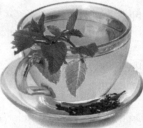

For a simple solution, which doesn't involve tablets at all, try adding fresh lemon juice to warm water and rinsing your mouth with it.

Cholesterol

Lemon pulp contains pectin, a type of soluble fiber that has been shown to help lower levels of LDL "bad" cholesterol. To get the cholesterol-lowering benefits of pectin, eat the whole lemon, not just the juice.

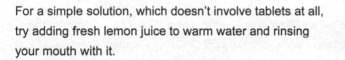

For a 1996 study published in the *Journal of Nutrition*, researchers fed rats either pectin or another type of fiber to examine the effect on cholesterol levels. Pectin was found to be one of the fibers that lowered average cholesterol levels. The authors of the study wrote:

"The addition of pectin to the diet resulted in lower serum and liver cholesterol concentrations."

Several studies have found that the flavonoids and rich vitamin C content of lemons may also help to lower cholesterol levels.

On flavonoids, the authors of a 1996 study published in the *Journal of Nutritional Biochemistry* wrote:

"Epidemiological studies show an inverse correlation between dietary flavonoid intake and mortality from coronary heart disease (CHD) which is explained in part by the inhibition of low density lipoprotein [LDL] oxidation and reduced platelet aggregability."

Clear skin

Sometimes we forget that the key to clear and beautiful skin starts with great nutrition. Thanks to the vitamin C in lemons, these little citrus fruits can help decrease wrinkles and blemishes. Vitamin C is a powerful antioxidant, and getting an ample amount in your diet can keep you looking and feeling youthful.

Researchers involved in a 2007 study published in the *American Journal of Clinical Nutrition* tested the effects of certain nutrients on the "skin-aging" of American women between the ages of 40 and 74. One of the nutrients tested was vitamin C. Regarding the effect of vitamin C on the skin, the study authors wrote:

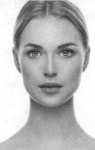

"Higher vitamin C intakes were associated with a lower likelihood of a wrinkled appearance... and senile dryness."

Lemons also help to push toxins from the body and support healthy liver function, which also keeps skin clear and supple.

Detox

Lemon juice helps to cleanse the liver by liquefying bile and dissolving uric acid. Your liver is vital to cleansing your blood, so keeping it as healthy and free of toxins as possible is essential. Furthermore, lemons can also help to cleanse toxins from your urinary tract, since they contain natural diuretic properties.

A 2005 study published in *BMC Pharmacology* found that hesperidin, a bioflavonoid present in citrus fruits, decreased chemically-induced oxidative stress levels in the liver and kidneys of rats. On their results, the study authors wrote:

"Our study demonstrated a protective effect of HDN [hesperidin] in CCl4 induced oxidative stress in rat liver and kidney. This protective effect of HDN can be correlated to its direct antioxidant effect."

Adding lemon juice to water or fresh green juices is an easy detox practice that you can incorporate into your daily diet.

Digestive health

Your body works hard to digest all that you put into it. Lemons help to flush away unwanted materials and toxins left from the digestive process. Because lemon juice is similar in atomic composition to digestive juices and saliva, it does a great job breaking down material and encouraging the liver to produce bile.

A 2011 study published in the journal *Chemico-Biological Interactions* found that the in vitro use of lemon essential oil, and its limonene component, "offered effective gastro-protection" against gastric ulcers.

Adding lemons to your diet may also help to relieve digestive disturbances such as bloating and indigestion.

Fatigue

Lemons, especially in the form of fresh lemon water, can help to bring about a fantastic energy boost. Not only is it hydrating—and we all know dehydration can lead to fatigue—it also helps to oxygenate your body. Additionally, it provides your body with the vitamins and minerals that it needs to perk up and function optimally.

A 2007 study published in the journal *Japanese Pharmacological Therapy* tested the effects of the citric acid found in lemon juice on the fatigue levels of 625 participants over a 28-day period. On their results, the study authors wrote:

"It… turned out that the drink containing lemon citric acid was useful for people frequently feeling fatigue."

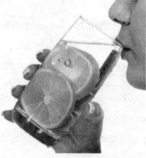

These yummy citrus fruits also helps to lift "brain fog," so when the afternoon yawns show up, sip on a glass of lemon water for a pick-me-up.

Fiber

Most people fall far short of the 20 to 38 grams of fiber recommended daily. Without proper fiber, however, you can easily become constipated or develop hemorrhoids. Consuming adequate fiber has also been shown to reduce the risk of developing health conditions such as diabetes, heart disease, and diverticulitis.

In fact, the *American Diabetes Association* includes lemons on their list of superfoods because of their high fiber content. In addition, the pectin fiber in lemons can help to curb cravings, thus helping you to keep your weight in check.

On the potential benefits of pectin for weight loss, the authors of a 1988 study published in the journal *Gastroenterology* wrote:

"As pectin induces satiety and delays gastric emptying in obese patients, it may be a useful adjuvant in the treatment of disorders of overeating."

Free radical fighter

As we've mentioned, vitamin C is a crucially important antioxidant for your body. The vitamin neutralizes free radicals both inside and outside of cells. Free radicals, which are byproducts of oxidative stress, are responsible for damaging cells and cellular membranes. If left unchecked, this damage can lead to inflammation, accelerated aging, and a host of chronic diseases.

Free radicals can also damage blood vessels and alter cholesterol so that it builds up on artery walls. Vitamin C helps prevent this buildup, and consequently helps to stop the progression of atherosclerosis and heart disease in diabetics.

On the protective effects of vitamin C against a variety of chronic conditions, the authors of a 1999 study published in *The American Journal of Clinical Nutrition* wrote:

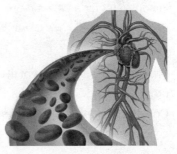

"Recent scientific evidence indicates that an increased intake of vitamin C is associated with a reduced risk of chronic diseases such as cancer, cardiovascular disease, and cataract."

The flavonoids found in lemons are linked to fighting free radicals and oxidative stress, as well. For a 1998 study published in the journal *Lipids*, researchers tested the role of certain flavonoids found in lemons for their ability to fight oxidative stress in diabetic rats. On their results, the researchers wrote:

"Crude flavonoids, eriocitrin, and hesperidin suppressed the oxidative stress in the diabetic rats. These results demonstrated that dietary lemon flavonoids of eriocitrin and hesperidin play a role as antioxidant in vivo."

Good source of potassium

We've already mentioned the role of potassium in potentially mitigating anxiety and depression, as well as in lowering blood pressure. However, this crucial mineral has many other functions. One is to balance out the sodium in the body, which is very important to kidney and cardiovascular health. It also helps to reduce the risk of kidney stones.

On the role of potassium in decreasing kidney stone risk, the authors of a 1993 study published in the *New England Journal of Medicine* wrote:

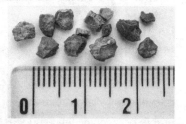

"Potassium intake and fluid intake were inversely related to the risk of kidney stones."

Potassium is also vital to the health of the nervous system, and getting a good amount of this mineral may help ease PMS symptoms in women.

Healthy feet

Lemon essential oil can help dissolve hardened patches of skin like corns and callouses. Use this essential oil directly on the hardened skin, but be careful not to get the oil on other areas, as it may be too strong in its undi-luted form for skin that is not hardened. In addition, it has aromatic and antiseptic properties and can be used to help relax tense foot muscles.

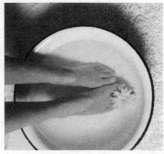

Also, try adding lemon juice to warm water for a healthy, relaxing foot bath.

Immune system booster

When cold and flu season arrives, it is a good idea to keep a bag of fresh lemons handy. The citric acid, bioflavonoids, vitamin C, calcium, pectin, and limonene found in lemons do a great job of boosting your immune system and keeping infections at bay.

On flavonoids, the authors of a 1996 study published in the *International Journal of Pharmacognosy* wrote:

"A variety of in vitro and in vivo experiments have shown that selected flavonoids possess antiallergic, anti-inflammatory, antiviral and antioxidant activities… a consid-erable body of evidence suggests that plant flavonoids may be health-promoting, disease-preventing dietary compounds."

If you do happen to catch a bug, sipping on warm lemon water may help you to recover quicker.

Increased iron absorption

Iron deficiency is certainly not uncommon, and can lead to anemia if left unchecked. Pairing foods high in vitamin C with those rich in iron will help the body to absorb more of the iron.

On the relationship between vitamin C and iron absorption, the authors of a 1989 study published in the *International Journal for Vitamin and Nutrition Research* state:

"The key role of ascorbic acid [vitamin C] for the absorption of dietary nonheme iron is generally accepted. The reasons for its action are twofold: (1) the prevention of the formation of insoluble and unabsorbable iron compounds and (2) the reduction of ferric to ferrous iron, which seems to be a requirement for the uptake of iron into the mucosal cells."

Try squeezing lemon juice onto a spinach salad, or enjoying hummus, which contains lemon juice and iron-rich chickpeas.

Insomnia

Insomnia, especially chronic insomnia, can be extremely damaging to your health, as sleep is so important for all of the body's systems to function properly. The tangy and sweet aroma of lemon essential oil has been found to be relaxing, and may help soothe you into restful sleep.

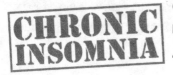

On lemons and insomnia, the authors of a 2009 study published by *ResearchGate* wrote:

"Insomnia is one of the most common sleep disorders around the world. Species of plants such as Citrus sinensis, Citrus limon [lemon], Ternstroemia pringlei, Ternstroemia sylvatica, Casimiroa edulis, Galphimia glauca and Cymbopogon citratus are traditionally and widely used in Mexico as sleep aids. The aim of this work was to evaluate the sedative effect of different extracts of these plants by using the exploratory cylinder model in mice."

Based on their research, the study authors concluded:

"Our results give evidence of the popular use of these medicinal plants as sleep aids."

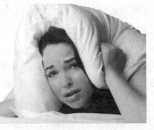

Along with using lemon essential oil for aromatherapy, sipping a cup of tea made with fresh lemons before bed may boost your Z's, as well.

Kidney stones

We've already covered that getting an ample amount of potassium, found in lemons, may help to prevent kidney stones. Additionally, when you don't have enough citrate in your urine, you are at an increased risk of developing kidney stones.

Eating lemons on a regular basis can help raise the citrate levels in your urine. A stone forms when calcium binds to oxalate or phosphate. However, citrate will bind to calcium, thus preventing it from binding to oxalate and phosphate to form stones.

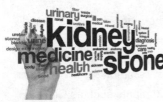

A 2007 study published in the journal *BMC Urology* examined the effects of lemon juice on calcium oxalate kidney stone formation (urolithiasis) in rats. In this study, the rats were given drinking water containing ethylene glycol (EG) and ammonium chloride (AC) in order to promote kidney stones.

The study authors wrote:

"This EG/AC-induced increase in kidney calcium levels was inhibited by the administration of lemon juice. Histology showed that rats treated with EG/AC alone had large deposits of calcium oxalate crystals in all parts of the kidney, and that such deposits were not present in rats also treated with either 100% or 75% lemon juice... These data suggest that lemon juice has a protective activity against urolithiasis."

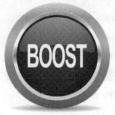

Mood and energy booster

Have you ever gotten up on the "wrong side of the bed"? If you are often lethargic and cranky in the morning, or at any time of the day for that matter, you may want to consider munching on a lemon.

Our energy comes from the atoms and molecules in our food. When positively charged atoms flood the digestive tract and mingle with those that are negatively charged, a positive reaction occurs.

Lemons contain more negatively charged ions than positive ions, which gives you a boost as the lemon enters your digestive tract. Just the scent of lemons alone can improve your mood and elevate your energy levels. As mentioned, lemons also promote clear thinking and help reduce anxiety and depression.

The authors of a 2009 study published in the journal *Aroma Research* wrote:

"The purpose of this paper is to analyze the psychological effect given to pre symptomatic depression by using the lemon and the yuzu essential oil as an olfactory stimulus.

POMS and Semantic Differential method were used for the psychological assessment. As a result, the depression feeling and the tension anxiety of [the] pre symptomatic depression group were reduced by the lemon essential oil in a short time."

Oxygen uptake helper

Lemons have a purer concentration of negatively charged ions than any other fruit. Pierce J. Howard, PhD, author of *The Owner's Manual for the Brain; Everyday Applications from Mind-Brain Research*, says, "Negative ions increase the flow of oxygen to the brain; resulting in higher alertness, decreased drowsiness, and more mental energy. They also may protect against germs in the air."

Possibly due to its potential effect of increasing oxygen to the brain, some research has found that aromatherapy with lemon essential oil may help boost attention and learning. The authors of a 2010 study published in *NeuroSciences* analyzed the effects of lemon aroma on rats and their ability to solve labyrinths. On their results, the authors wrote:

"Our results indicate that the lemon aroma may have some effects on learning. The findings obtained from this study are consistent with the findings of similar research on the behavioral properties of the lemon aroma."

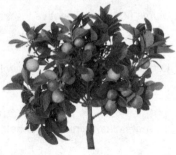

The first man to reach the top of Mount Everest, Sir Edmund Hillary, said that he attributed much of his success to lemons!

LEMON FACT: One lemon tree can produce up to 600 pounds of lemons in a year. If you live in an area where you can grow a lemon tree, why not plant one or two!

pH balancer

Lemons are considered one of the most alkalizing foods you can eat. This may seem counterintuitive, as they are acidic on their own. However, in the body, lemons have an alkalizing effect; the citric acid does not create acidity once it has been metabolized.

The minerals in lemons actually help to alkalize the blood. Most people are too acidic, and lemons reduce overall acidity, drawing uric acid from the joints. This may reduce the joint pain and inflammation which many people feel.

Regarding the alkalizing effects of lemons, the authors of a 2015 study published in *Annals of the Rheumatic Diseases* wrote:

"Lemon juice stimulates the formation of calcium carbonate released by the pancreas and aids in alkalization of the blood and urine, neutralizing acids such as uric acid."

The researchers involved in this study tested the ability of lemon juice to reduce uric acid levels in gout patients. On their results, the authors wrote:

"In this study all individuals given lemon water showed a reduction in SUA [serum uric acid], improvement of serum creatinine and GFR [glomerular filtration rate, a test of kidney functionality] as well as urine alkalization after 6 weeks of lemon water. Lemon water may be a useful adjuvant in the treatment of patients with gout."

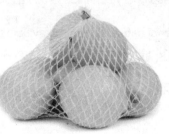

Reduce inflammation

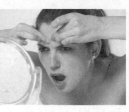

As discussed earlier, lemons can help to decrease the body's acidity and restore healthy pH. This, along with the many antioxidant compounds found in lemons, can help reduce inflammation throughout the body.

The authors of a 2007 study published in the journal *Food Science* tested the anti-inflammatory powers of citrus limonoids on mouse subjects. On their results, the authors wrote:

> *"Limonoids from citrus fruits have potent anti-inflammation and analgesic effect."*

Reducing systemic inflammation is vital to your overall health, as inflammation has been found at the root of many chronic conditions, including a host of autoimmune illnesses, as well as diabetes and heart disease.

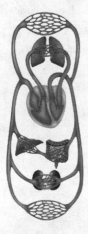

Respiratory conditions

The vitamin C in lemons can aid in the healing of all sorts of illnesses. In particular, lemon may provide some relief to sufferers of respiratory conditions such as asthma.

The antibacterial nature of lemon may help to fight respiratory infections. In a 2014 study published in *Pharmaceutical Sciences*, honey and lemon were tested for their ability to combat bacteria derived from respiratory tract infections. The study authors wrote:

"Excellent antibacterial activity was observed with lemon, honey and lemon mixture… Better killing of the bacteria isolates on exposure to honey and lemon was observed with lemon and honey/lemon mixture than the honey alone… This study justifies the use of honey and lemon separately and in mixture as an alternative medicine by the populace in the treatment of respiratory tract infections."

Soothe chapped lips

Rubbing fresh lemon juice onto puckered lips at night, then rinsing it off in the morning, is a great way to exfoliate dead skin and soften the lips. As an added bonus, your lipstick will go on more smoothly.

Stronger nails

Go to any pharmacy and you'll see a number of nail-strengthening products, however, these are often made from harsh chemicals. Combining lemon juice with olive oil and using the mixture as a nail soak is a natural alternative that can help to condition brittle nails. This easy soak can also help to whiten yellowed nails.

What Lemons Can Do for Your Home and Beauty

Besides their many benefits to your health, lemons are also great to have around your home—and as an essential part of your beauty regimen—for a number of reasons:

Berry stain remover

Berries are a delicious and nutritious treat, and it's so much fun to go pick them yourself. If you find that your fingers become stained from the berries (and they will if you pick enough), you will also find that regular soap and water will not come close to removing the stains. However, lemons offer a simple solution.

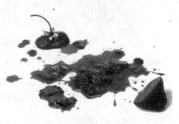

Just pour a little undiluted lemon juice on your hands, wait a few minutes, and wash with warm soapy water. Repeat until your hands are stain-free—it shouldn't take more than a couple of washes.

Breath freshener

For long-lasting fresh breath, rinse with straight lemon juice. Rather than spitting the juice out, swallow it. Citric acid, found in lemon juice, will alter the pH level in your mouth, killing the bacteria that cause breath odor. Rinse your mouth and teeth thoroughly with water after the lemon juice, as prolonged exposure to citric acid can damage tooth enamel.

Clean and whiten nails

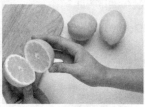

Whether you dig in the dirt a lot, have yellow stains from nail polish, or have dull and listless nails, lemon juice is just what you need. Lemons contain natural bleaching power that can restore your nails to a vivid white.

Fill a bowl halfway with fresh lemon juice. Place your nails in the juice for about fifteen minutes. Use a soft brush, or a toothbrush, to gently scrub the yellow from your nails. Rinse your hands with lukewarm water and apply a thin coat of coconut oil. Do this daily until your nail color has been restored.

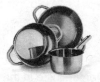

Clean brass and chrome

Does your brass or chrome need a pick-me-up? If so, let lemons do the work for you. You can easily make a paste with lemon juice and baking soda. Just mix enough of each to make the consistency of toothpaste. Apply the mixture to your brass or chrome and let it sit for about five minutes. Wash it off with warm water, then dry and polish with a clean cloth.

You can also clean your kitchen sink with this mixture, and the bonus is that it smells amazingly fresh. It will work to remove mineral deposits, as well.

Cutting board refresher

No matter how clean you try to keep your cutting boards, it is inevitable that they will capture the odors of the foods that you cut on them. After each use, cut a lemon in half and rub the cutting board down. You can also pour some lemon juice in a small spray bottle and spritz the board after each use. Rinse well and allow the board to air dry.

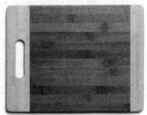

Dandruff fighter

Many people are plagued with dandruff, and tirelessly seek relief. Thankfully, there is a very easy way to ease dandruff using lemon juice. Massage two tablespoons of lemon juice into your scalp and rinse with water. Next, stir one teaspoon of lemon juice into a cup of water and rinse your hair with it—repeat this until you see an improvement in your dandruff.

Healthy skin

Lemon juice can be used to ease the pain of sunburn, other minor burns, and bee stings, and it may help minimize scars from old burns. It can also be used to help relieve eczema. In addition, it has anti-aging properties, and can be used to help remove blackheads.

To use as an acne treatment, pour a small amount of lemon juice onto a cotton ball, then apply to the area of concern before going to bed. Rinse off the lemon juice in the morning.

Insect repellant

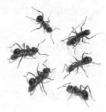

If you have small children or pets, you may be wary of using a chemical treatment for insects that decide to take up residence in your home. To keep ants and other insects out, spray a little lemon juice on door thresholds and window sills. If you can see where the ants, or other unwanted guests, are coming from, squeeze a little juice into the holes or cracks.

You can also cut up small pieces of lemon and place them outside of doors. To deter roaches and fleas, mix the juice of four lemons, and the rinds, with a half gallon of water, and wash your floors with the mixture.

Lighten age spots

Age spots, also known as liver spots, are harmless spots that generally appear in people over 50. They can sometimes be the result of sun exposure. While they are harmless, many people find them unsightly. If you are one of these people, you can lighten these spots naturally with lemon.

Simply apply some fresh lemon juice to the dark area (a spray bottle works well), and let it sit on the spot for about fifteen minutes before rinsing it off. Keep this up daily and you will see the spot lighten in no time.

Make soggy lettuce firm

Do you hate soggy lettuce, and often find yourself throwing it out? Before you do, try this: Add the juice of half a lemon to a bowl of cold water and place the soggy lettuce in the bowl. Refrigerate for one hour. You will be amazed at what happens to your limp lettuce. Just take the leaves out of the lemon juice mixture and dry them off before using in your salad.

Natural hair highlights

Do you dream of beautiful hair highlights but dread using heavy chemicals? Using lemon juice for lightening your hair is a wonderful way to get lovely highlights without exposing yourself to toxins. Mix one-quarter of a cup of lemon juice with three-quarters of a cup of water, and use this mixture to rinse your hair. After you rinse, sit in the sun until your hair dries. Repeat this once daily for up to a week until you see the desired effect.

Warm Lemon Water: Super Simple Health Tonic

Ayurvedic philosophy states that the choices that we make each day can either build us up or make us more susceptible to life-destroying disease.

Because we are exposed to so many environmental toxins, from what we breathe in to what we put on our skin—in addition to the damaging impact of our Western diet—our bodies can quickly shift into toxic overdrive.

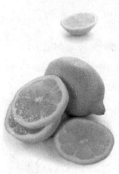

While we sleep each night, our bodies continue to work to rebalance, heal, repair, restore, and revitalize us, so that we can have ample energy to face the next day. If you knew that there was one simple, inexpensive thing you could do each day to aid your body in building up your health and clear away toxins, would you do it?

Consuming a cup of warm lemon water upon rising is one small change that can make a dramatic impact on how our bodies function. If this seems too simple to be true, we invite you to read on.

The Alternative Daily

The health promoting benefits of lemons are old news. For centuries, it has been known that lemons contain powerful antibacterial, antiviral, and immune boosting components. We know that lemons are a great digestive aid and liver cleanser.

As mentioned, lemons contain citric acid, magnesium, bioflavonoids, vitamin C, pectin, calcium, and limonene, which supercharge our immunity so that our bodies can fight infection. Drinking lemon water every morning can give your body the boost it may need to keep you as healthy as possible.

How to Make Warm Lemon Water

While it is not rocket science, making warm lemon water involves paying particular attention to a couple of things. The water you use should be purified and lukewarm. Don't make the water super hot, and avoid cold water. It is hard on the body, especially first thing in the morning, to ask it to process ice-cold water, so make sure you get the temperature right.

Always use fresh, organic lemons in your water—never bottled lemon juice. Squeeze the juice of half a lemon into a glass of warm water. Be sure to drink the lemon water before you eat anything.

Kicking off your morning with warm lemon water is a great way to provide your body with the many health benefits of lemons, detailed earlier in this book. Along with being a perfect morning tonic, warm lemon water also makes a nice pre-workout drink.

More on Lemons and Weight Loss

The notion that tangy, delicious lemons can help with weight loss may seem too good to be true. However, they really can help quite a bit. The following are a few ways that lemons can potentially help you maintain a healthy weight.

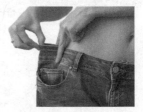

A low-sugar alternative

Of course, eating lemons alone is not a magic weight loss solution. But if you choose to drink lemon water instead of soda or coffee with sugar, it can certainly support your weight loss goals.

Better digestion

Lemons support digestive health and can have a mild diuretic effect, so consuming them can help you to shed some water weight. While this is, of course, not the same as losing body fat, it is a good start and can certainly help you to feel lighter and less bloated.

Improved metabolism

Lemons are rich in potassium, which is important for healthy metabolic functioning. While it's a leap to say that lemons will give you a super-charged metabolism, including lemons as part of a healthy diet can help to maintain the kind of metabolic efficiency you want when you're trying to lose weight.

Curb cravings

Some anecdotal reports suggest that lemon water can help satiate food cravings. While we may sometimes crave healthy foods as a result of our bodies needing a certain nutrient, many of us develop emotional fixations around certain foods—or just around eating in general—that are not necessarily related to our body's nutritional needs.

When this is the case, drinking lemon water can help satisfy the desire to consume something.

Mineral absorption

It is thought that lemons may help with the absorption of certain minerals. If we're not absorbing sufficient nutrients, we're more likely to continue experiencing cravings, regardless of how many calories we're consuming. While this is an indirect connection, any healthy food that can help to curb cravings is potentially beneficial when you're trying to lose weight.

Simply drinking lemon water is not enough to help you achieve significant weight loss, but it is a beneficial addition to a healthy diet and exercise plan. Also, because of their low calorie content and nutrient density, there's very little to lose by upping your lemon intake—and much to gain.

More on Lemons and Cancer

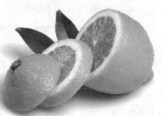

Sometimes, the greatest assets to your health are also the simplest. Lemons, as well as other citrus fruits, provide a diverse and plentiful array of benefits to the body. Eating organic citrus fruits and drinking freshly squeezed citrus juices can give your skin a healthy glow, boost your immune system, and, according to some studies, could even help fight a variety of cancers.

One of the best known health properties of citrus fruits such as lemons is their high vitamin C content. As we've mentioned, vitamin C is a powerful antioxidant, which aids the immune system in all of its disease-fighting functions. Lemons also contain flavonoids, which increase the potency of vitamin C, reduce bodily inflammation, improve circulation, and help regulate blood pressure.

Lemons also aid in the detoxification of the liver by stimulating natural liver enzymes, which helps keep your circulatory system, and your skin, clear. The electrolytes found in lemons help keep your body hydrated and functioning optimally.

Lab studies of the limonoids and citrus pectins found in lemons have shown that these compounds can help slow the growth of cancer cells, keep them from spreading, and also in some cases destroy the cancer cells themselves. Studies have found that limonoids promote cytotoxicity to breast, colon, liver, and pancreatic cancers, as well as to leukemia and neuroblastoma.

In one study, which set out to test the effect of limonoids on breast cancer cells, nine different limonoids were extracted from dried lemon seeds. Seven of these nine limonoids showed significant cytotoxicity against ER+ breast cancer cells. Four of the nine limonoids were cytotoxic to ER- breast cancer cells, and decreased their growth by approximately 44 percent. The most potent of the limonoids was limonin glucoside, which is the most prevalent limonoid in citrus juices.

Another recent case-control study, performed in Europe, found that four or more 150-gram portions of citrus fruits per week decreased the risk of throat cancer by 58 percent, oral/pharyngeal cancer by 53 percent, and stomach cancer by 31 percent.

Limonoids are found in the juices, pulp, and peels of all citrus fruits. If you include pulp when juicing your lemons, oranges, and grapefruits, you will increase your intake of limonoid gluco- sides significantly. Approximately 75 grams of citrus fruits and juices per day is recommended to help aid your body in natural cancer prevention.

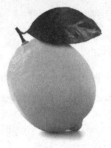

Lemon Essential Oil

Lemon essential oil, made by cold-pressing lemon rinds, is a great way to get many of the benefits of lemon, as it basically concentrates its goodness into one tiny, portable bottle. Unlike fresh lemons, it does not go bad, and it can do in a pinch if you find that you don't have any whole fresh lemons.

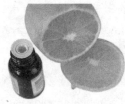

Due to its concentrated nature, lemon essential oil has a host of versatile uses. The following are just 13 of the hundreds out there:

Add some natural highlights

We mentioned earlier that fresh lemon, combined with sunshine, can help lighten your hair. This works with lemon essential oil, as well. If there's ample sunshine where you live, and you're seeking some natural blonde highlights, apply lemon essential oil to your hair in streaks or strands, then go out in the sun for a few minutes.

Banish nail fungus

Applying undiluted lemon essential oil to fingernail or toenail fungus throughout the day may help to clear it up.

Boost your spirits

A little bit of aromatherapy with lemon essential oil, either circulated through the room in a diffuser, or applied to pressure points, can improve your mood.

Clean the kitchen

Just as you can use fresh lemons to clean your home, you can use lemon essential oil, too. In an empty spray bottle (preferably glass), combine one part water with one part white vinegar. Add about six or seven drops of lemon essential oil, and shake. This multipurpose spray is great for cleaning counters, tables, chairs, your fridge, and your sink. Simple and chemical-free.

Degrease oily hair

Adding a drop of lemon essential oil to a handful of your regular, organic shampoo can help cut the grease and leave your hair feeling healthy. For very long or thick hair, use two drops.

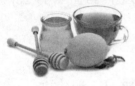

Ease congestion

Rubbing lemon essential oil on your throat may help when you feel stuffed up. You can also add a couple of drops of food-grade lemon essential oil to a cup of herbal tea.

Enhance your focus

Speaking of aromatherapy, did you know that the scent of lemon can improve cognitive clarity so that you can zero in on the task at hand? Try a dab on your temples next time you're in a bind at the office.

Exfoliate your skin

To make a great exfoliating scrub, combine oatmeal, raw honey, and a bit of water to make a paste. Add a few drops of lemon essential oil, mix, and rub on your face in a gentle circular motion. Wait about five minutes, then rinse and wash your face with a gentle organic soap.

Freshen your breath

If your breath is less than fresh, add a few drops of food-grade lemon essential oil to a glass of warm water, and gargle. You can also freshen your toothbrush with this oil: a drop or so on a weekly basis will keep bad breath at bay, and keep pathogens off your brush.

Help heal bug bites

Dabbing a bit of lemon essential oil onto bug bites and bee stings can help to prevent infection, and may help heal the bite faster.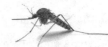

Kick cold sores to the curb

Use a cotton swab to dab lemon essential oil onto a cold sore up to three times per day. This promotes healing, and may help make that scaly patch disappear.

Speed digestion

If you ate something a bit too heavy, or your digestion is just working too slowly, try gently massaging some lemon essential oil, blended with some organic coconut oil, onto your tummy.

Soothe a sore throat

Along with adding a couple of drops in your herbal tea throughout the day, you can mix a drop of lemon essential oil into a warm salt-water gargle.

As you can see, lemon essential oil has many of the same benefits as a fresh lemon—with a few variations here and there. It can be especially helpful when traveling or at work, so be sure to pack a bottle in your purse or briefcase!

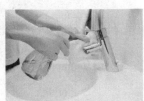

Lemons and Dogs

The American Society for the Prevention of Cruelty to Animals states that citrus fruit may be harmful to dogs. According to their report, the pith (fiber), the seeds, and the peel can cause the most damage. Eaten in large quantities, lemons may cause photosensitivity issues, lethargy, or digestive issues (such as vomiting or diarrhea), and dogs may become dehydrated as a result of this reaction.

Just like in humans, eating too much citrus can be painful and have undesirable side effects for dogs. Grapefruit is the most dangerous, and should not be given to our canine friends.

However, as long as you only give your dog lemon in small quantities, and just give them the juice or a lemon extract, it is far from toxic. On the contrary, lemon may actually provide numerous health benefits to your pet.

The vitamin needs of dogs

Just like humans, dogs need a wide variety of vitamins to function at optimal levels. According to research collected by *The Bark* magazine, dogs need the following nutrients in their diet:

- Vitamin A
- Vitamin D

The Alternative Daily

- Vitamin E
- Vitamin C
- Vitamin K
- B vitamins
- Silicone
- Magnesium
- Selenium
- Molybdenum
- Fluorine
- Cobalt
- Manganese
- Chromium
- Copper
- Iodine
- Iron
- Sulfur
- Zinc
- Calcium
- Potassium
- Sodium
- Chloride
- Phosphorous

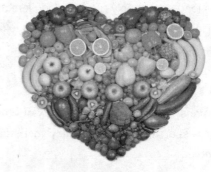

Of these essential nutrients, lemons provide a significant amount of vitamin C, B vitamins, vitamin E, copper, magnesium, manganese, phosphorous, and potassium. Lemon juice alone can provide many of the vital nutrients that a dog needs each day.

Can't dogs make their own vitamin C?

Most health experts agree that dogs can make their own vitamin C—they can synthesize the nutrient from a variety of sources. However, evidence suggests that dogs that do not routinely consume a source of vitamin C may be more susceptible to health problems.

A study from 1942 examined the effects of vitamin C on dogs with skin diseases. The study authors found that dogs who had skin diseases were likely to have lower levels of vitamin C than dogs with healthy skin. Dogs who had fevers and dogs pushed to physical capacity (such as those running long distances at top speeds) had low blood levels of vitamin C. This study found that stress is a depleting factor for a dog's vitamin C levels. The more stressed the dog, the lower the vitamin C level in their blood.

In 1965, Wendell O. Belfield, DVM, experimented with the use of vitamin C supplementation on dogs with health problems, based on the findings from the earlier study. During his vet practice, he experimented with using large doses of vitamin C to treat common health issues in dogs, such as distemper. Just like in humans, the doses of vitamin C were able to help dogs fight their health problems.

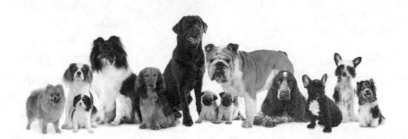

According to a 1996 book titled *Encyclopedia of Nutritional Supplements*, vitamin C is essential for building the immune system because it is able to increase the effectiveness of white blood cells. Vitamin C also encourages the growth of interferon cells and antibodies, which fight cell mutation and infection. Based on these findings, small doses of lemon may not only be safe for dogs to consume, but may actually boost their overall health.

Possible health benefits of lemon for dogs

There are multiple breeds of dogs, and not all dogs will respond to lemon in the same way. Additionally, most of the remedies on this list have not been studied in a lab setting, which means there is no scientific backing for their use. However, based on the science of how vitamin C works in humans, who are similar to dogs in many ways, the following uses for vitamin C may be beneficial to your dog's health:

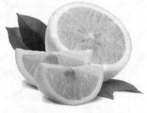

Anti-aging and cancer-fighting properties

Lemons contain high levels of antioxidants. Antioxidants not only fight the oxidation of cells, which causes signs of aging, but also fight against the growth and spread of cancer cells. A daily dose of lemon, containing 22 antioxidants, could help prevent the development of cancer in your best friend.

Antibacterial effects

Lemons are antibacterial, which can be beneficial both for the health of your dog's intestines and for your dog's breath. A daily intake of lemon water could help fight bad breath, while preventing tooth decay at the same time.

Digestive regulator

Although large doses of lemon juice can have a negative effect on the stomach and intestines, the right dose can have a beneficial effect. The antibacterial properties in lemons can help eliminate unwanted bacteria from the intestines and bring balance back to your pet's digestive system. Lemons may also be able to prevent your dog from getting worms.

Ear infections

If your dog gets frequent ear infections, a gentle wash of lemon water can help fight the infection and keep it from getting worse. If you attempt this remedy, never pour water directly into your dog's ears, as this can make the infection worse. Rather, use a damp cloth to rub a dollop of lemon oil or a lemon-juice-infused rag around the outside of your dog's ear and into the visible part of the ear canal.

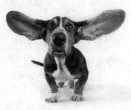

Immune system booster

According to the studies mentioned above, vitamin C is beneficial in boosting the immune system in dogs as well as humans. Vitamin C is essential for supporting the effectiveness of white blood cells in fighting off invaders and common ailments.

Nutrient harvester

Vitamin C helps boost the absorption rate of other vitamins that are essential to your dog's health, such as vitamin B3, calcium, vitamin E and glutathione.

Healthy bones and teeth

As mentioned above, lemon juice not only fights plaque and bacteria in the mouth, but it can also boost the absorption of other nutrients that your dog needs to build strong teeth and bones, such as calcium. Vitamin C is one of the most beneficial nutrients for your dog's dental health.

Insect repellant

Mosquitoes and other insects do not like the flavor of lemon or lemon oil. Applying lemon topically to your dog's fur can help deter insect bites.

How to give lemon to dogs

As stated earlier, avoid giving your dog large doses of lemon at once, and don't give him or her the fiber, seeds, or peel of a lemon. This could result in unwanted side effects and pain for your dog. Instead, add lemon juice or lemon essential oil to your dog's daily routine. (Lemon essential oil should only be used topically.)

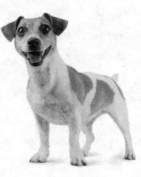

For questions on how specific breeds will respond to lemon, it may be wise to have a conversation with your vet—just to be safe.

Suggested doses

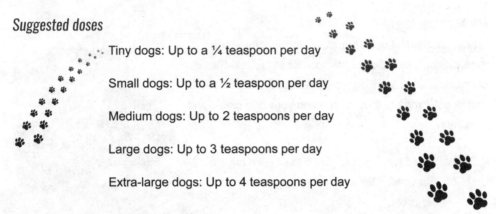

Tiny dogs: Up to a ¼ teaspoon per day

Small dogs: Up to a ½ teaspoon per day

Medium dogs: Up to 2 teaspoons per day

Large dogs: Up to 3 teaspoons per day

Extra-large dogs: Up to 4 teaspoons per day

Try these serving ideas for your dog:

- Mix a small amount of fresh lemon juice into your dog's water bowl.

- Squeeze some fresh lemon juice over your dog's food.

- Use lemon essential oil topically on your dog's skin, or in topical recipes.

Beneficial Lemon Recipes for Dogs

Lemon Flea Spray/ Insect Repellant

- Cut up two lemons into thin slices.

- Place the lemons in a pot with two cups of water.

- Boil the lemon slices for about five minutes.

- Allow the lemon slices to steep in the water overnight.

The next day, place the lemon water (with the lemons removed) into a spray bottle and spray on your dog's fur to help eliminate fleas.

Lemon Shampoo

Many commercial dog shampoos contain unhealthy ingredients. Instead of exposing your pet to toxic chemicals, you can make your own lemon shampoo that is safe and effective at keeping your dog clean and healthy.

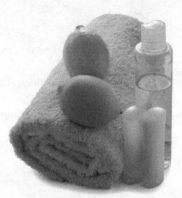

- Steep two bags of green tea in two cups of hot water. Discard the tea bags once the water cools.

- Add the juice of one lemon.

- Add five tablespoons of unfiltered apple cider vinegar.

- Allow the mixture to steep overnight, then the following day, it will be ready for use.

Although this mixture may seem like it would not be an effective cleaner, you may be surprised at how well it works. When using this shampoo, keep it out of your dog's eyes. You can adjust the recipe based on how large your dog is. It should keep for about a week before it starts to go bad.

Lemon Yogurt

Yogurt is safe for dogs to eat, and it can help provide bacterial balance in their intestines—just like in humans. Add about a quarter of a teaspoon of lemon to your dog's yogurt before serving it to him or her for a tasty, healthy treat.

Lemon Bacon Treats

These lemony treats will make your dog smile.

Ingredients:

- 1 ½ cups organic rice flour
- 1 ½ cups wheat germ
- 2 free-range eggs
- 1 cup homemade chicken broth
- 1 cup bacon fat
- 1 cup oatmeal
- 2 tablespoons fresh lemon juice

Instructions:

1. Preheat the oven to 350°F.

2. Combine all the ingredients together to form a dough. Roll out the dough to a half-inch thickness and cut out pieces with a cookie cutter. Bake for 20 minutes or until lightly browned. Allow the cookies to cool and harden before giving them to your dog.

Growing Lemons

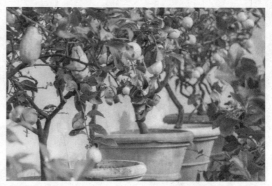

Lemons, like other fruits in the citrus family, prefer subtropical climates and thrive in the heat. The U.S. Department of Agriculture recommends growing lemons in zones 9 through 11. Although lemons can be grown in regions outside of the recommended zones, be aware that fruit production will likely be less than optimal as a reflection of the growing conditions. Citrus trees, in general, are best grown between sea level and 2,450 feet in the subtropics, and between sea level and 5,250 feet in the tropics.

Lemon trees thrive in temperatures ranging from 77 to 86 degrees Fahrenheit, although they can tolerate higher temperatures. For example, lemon trees are often grown in California, where temperatures can exceed 100 degrees Fahrenheit. Lemons are more sensitive to cold temperatures than other citrus varieties. The fruit is killed within 30 minutes if the temperature drops to 28 degrees Fahrenheit or lower. The trees can become inactive at 55 degrees Fahrenheit.

Lemon trees are able to withstand poor and slightly acidic soils, and in this respect, they are relatively hardy. They do, however, prefer well-drained soils. Lemon trees require weekly deep watering. They also thrive when raised slightly above the ground. It is best to plant them shallower than the length of the root ball, and it is a good idea to add mulch to retain the moisture. Pruning can help lemon trees maintain their shape and height.

If you do not live in a climate conducive to planting lemons outside, you can grow lemons indoors—they can be easily maintained as a potted plant. They will, however, need to be potted in an area that will allow them to grow three to five feet. When potted indoors they will need well-drained, slightly acidic soil.

Lemons require a lot of sunlight, therefore plants kept inside may need fluorescent lighting during the winter months. During summer months, it is recommended to place your potted trees outside so that they can receive direct sunlight, which can increase their fruit production. Fruits can take six to eight months to ripen.

Tips & Techniques

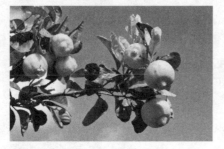

There are a variety of tips and tricks to help you with regards to growing, harvesting, and ripening your lemons. For instance, purchasing a one-year-old nursery tree that is already established means it will grow at a faster rate. To plant the tree, dig up any grass and raise the plant bed for better drainage. Fertilize the tree with a natural fertilizer that contains nitrogen for the first year, from spring to summer months.

Water the tree as needed, and be sure to water more frequently during droughts or in dry climates. Prune as needed to maintain proper growth.

You can grow lemons organically by purchasing an organic nursery tree or seeds, ensuring good drainage, fertilizing the soil with organic material, and providing your tree with a decent amount of sunlight and warmth. To grow a tree from organic seeds, it is best to use organic soil so as not to contaminate the lemons with inorganic material, which can hinder their growth. Non-organic lemons cannot produce new trees from their seeds. However, it is possible to germinate the seeds of organic lemons.

If you are tight on space or live in a less-than-ideal climate for lemons, Meyer lemons might be your best option, due to their size. These little lemons are ideal for growing in containers.

Lemons require 10 to 14 hours of direct sunlight during the sprouting stage. FIrst, fill your container with premoisturized soil, leaving an inch below the rim of the pot or container. Remove the seeds from the lemon. Do not allow the seeds to dry, as they need moisture to germinate. Plant your seeds roughly half an inch below the surface.

Cover the container with a breathable plastic to retain heat and moisture. Place the container in a warm place for the next few days. Keep a watchful eye, and don't let the soil dry out completely during the germination period. If you are successful, you will notice sprouts within two weeks. Once sprouts emerge, remove the plastic and place the container in direct sunlight.

Occasionally a tree may struggle to flourish. The following are some tips on how to troubleshoot problems: To revive a dying citrus tree, first determine what is causing it to die. If the tree needs more water, ensure that the drainage is adequate, then water it more frequently. Dig composted horse or cow manure, if available, and apply it at the base of the tree to encourage good drainage. If weeds are the problem, pull up the weeds and surrounding grass and add mulch to prevent weed growth.

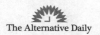

If your tree has a fungus growth, apply a natural fungicide. Inspect your tree for any insect infestation that could be causing it to die, and treat it for any diseases it may have. Remove shrubs nearby that could be preventing your tree from receiving adequate sunlight. Remember, lemon trees need at least eight hours of direct sunlight each day.

Lemons cannot effectively be ripened at home—so make sure you get the tree into the sun for the fruit to ripen. Placing ripe lemons in a cool environment or a refrigerator can prevent them from rotting before you have the chance to enjoy them.

Wrapping it up

There you have it, lemons can surely brighten your day, keep your house clean, help you look and feel your best, and keep your furry friends healthy. We hope you have enjoyed this brief look at one of nature's most alluring little fruits.

This page intentionally left blank.

67 Ways to Use Lemons Every Day...

Recipes for Health, Beauty and Home!

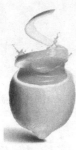

Lemons have so many amazing properties - start taking advantage of this amazing fruit today!

In this book you will discover some of the lemon's best uses. The book is grouped into four different categories: beauty, home, health & wellness and just for fun. The recipes use whole lemons, lemon juice, lemon peels and lemon essential oil.

Stock up the next time you see a special on lemons at the supermarket — you can squeeze the juice and then freeze it in ice cube-sized portions for easy use! You can also save already-squeezed lemons and freeze them for easier zesting.

Before we begin, however, a word of caution: lemons, like most other cultivated fruits, are often sprayed with harmful chemicals and pesticides to ensure they grow up imperfection-free. For this reason, it's always

best to choose **organic lemons** wherever possible. If your supermarket doesn't stock any or the price is prohibitive, that's okay — just keep in mind that the skin is where the highest concentration of these chemicals is found. You should avoid consuming lemon skin directly and any liquids that come into contact with those skins as much as you can if you don't choose organic. Don't fret too much, though!

Read on to enjoy all of the wonderful benefits of natural lemons!

Lemon Recipes For Beauty

Once you start to look into conventional beauty products, it's appalling how many toxic chemicals we apply to our skin and hair on a daily basis. These beauty products claim to nourish our complexion, fortify our hair and strengthen our nails, when really they're introducing toxins into our system and undermining our beauty from the inside out.

Sure, you can shop around and seek out "clean" products, which have less nasty ingredients, but the best thing you can do

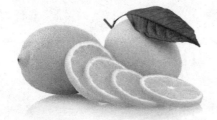

for your health and beauty routine is to get back to basics. These natural lemon-based solutions provide just that: the natural nurturing powers of the lemon in conjunction with other wholesome ingredients provide a truly guilt-free beauty treatment.

Recipe #1:
Lemon Yogurt Face Mask

This gentle mask combines the antibacterial properties of lemons and raw honey with the nurturing and brightening effects of yogurt. It's easy to make, and chances are you've already got all the required ingredients sitting around in your kitchen!

Ingredients:

- 1 tbsp lemon juice, freshly squeezed
- 1/4 cup plain Greek yogurt
- 1 tbsp raw honey

Equipment:

- Small bowl
- Spoon

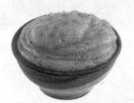

Instructions:

1. Mix the ingredients together in a small bowl.

2. Dampen face with warm water to open the pores.

3. Apply mask to face and let sit for 10 minutes.

4. Rinse with warm water.

Recipe #2:
Good Morning Face Scrub

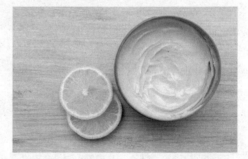

Ditch the toner and take a break from layering on the makeup with this natural, wholesome alternative. This face scrub will cleanse your pores, freshen your complexion and really brighten up your morning. Use this every day to keep your skin looking young and vibrant, and ensure you don't need to rely on makeup to look your best.

67 Ways to Use Lemons Every Day...
Recipes for Health, Beauty and Home!

Ingredients:

- 2 tbsp raw honey
- 1 tbsp coconut sugar crystals
- 1/4 lemon, freshly squeezed juice

Equipment:

- Small glass container
- Spoon

Instructions:

1. Mix the ingredients together in a small glass container. This recipe yields 4 or 5 uses.

2. Moisten skin with warm water, then scrub gently with the mixture.

3. Leave on for a few minutes, then rinse and pat dry.

Recipe #3:
Simple DIY Cuticle Cream

The daily rigors of life can really take a toll on your cuticles. The dry, recirculated air of your apartment during winter, repeatedly dunking your hands in hot water to wash the dishes, or just not treating your digits as well as you should will all conspire to undermine your cuticles and make them something of a hindrance.

This super simple homemade cream will give your cuticles some much-needed love. They'll be hydrated and supple in no time!

Ingredients:

- 1/2 cup pure shea butter
- 1 tsp extra virgin olive oil
- 1/2 cup freshly squeezed lemon juice

Instructions:

1. In a saucepan over low heat, gently warm the shea butter until it becomes liquid, stirring constantly. Remove from heat.

2. Transfer the shea butter to a small glass bowl, then add in the olive oil and lemon juice. Mix until all ingredients are combined and formed a creamy texture.

3. Store the cuticle cream in an airtight glass container and apply to your cuticles as needed.

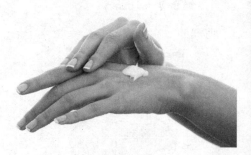

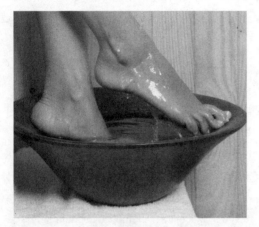

Recipe #4:
Easy At-Home Foot Soak

Considering the pivotal role feet play in getting us from A to B, they are surprisingly under-appreciated. Pounding the pavement and shoving our feet into tight, unforgiving shoes every day can leave them in a sorry state. They may even get to the point where you're embarrassed to take your socks off or wear flip flops on a hot day.

Luckily, we have just the thing — and it doesn't require spending a pile of money at the spa or on fancy foot treatments. This foot soak will have your feet looking fabulous once more, helping to banish rough skin and keep them nice and supple for a fraction of the cost!

Ingredients:

- 10 cups hot water
- 1 cup raw apple cider vinegar
- 1/2 cup salt
- 2 lemons, freshly squeezed

Equipment:

- Large bowl, bucket or basin

Instructions:

1. Combine ingredients in the large container.

2. Soak feet for 15 minutes, then pat dry. Follow with a scrub (see recipe #5).

Recipe #5:
Sweet Feet Moisturizing Scrub

Give your feet some long overdue TLC with this moisturizing foot scrub. It works just as well as pricey store-bought scrubs, but it costs a whole lot less to make and it's completely natural, so you know there's no toxic ingredients in there. This sweet foot scrub works wonders when used after recipe #4.

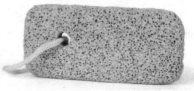

Ingredients:

- 1/2 cup brown sugar
- 2 tbsp olive oil
- 1/2 lemon, freshly squeezed

Equipment:

- Small bowl
- Spoon

Instructions:

1. Mix ingredients together in a small bowl.
2. Apply to feet and any other rough skin areas that need to be exfoliated.
3. Massage generously, then rinse and pat dry.

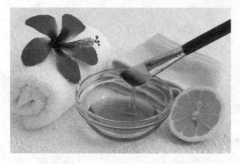

Recipe #6:
Lemon Olive Oil Face Mask

Try this moisturizing and nourishing recipe for combination skin. It will cleanse, tone and tighten the skin on your face.

Ingredients:

- 1 tsp olive oil
- A few drops fresh lemon juice
- 1/2 cup cooked instant oatmeal (cooled)
- 1 egg white

Equipment:

- Mixing bowl

Instructions:

1. Mix olive oil, lemon juice, oatmeal and egg white until smooth.
2. Spread on your face and neck. Leave on for 15 to 30 minutes.
3. Rinse with lukewarm water. Follow with your favorite non-toxic facial moisturizer if needed. You may find that your skin feels great after this mask and doesn't need anything else.

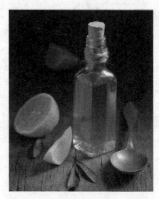

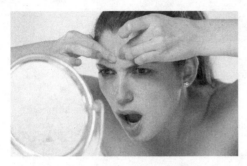

Instructions:

1. Cut a lemon in half, squeeze or smear some raw honey on it and add a light dusting of sugar on top.

2. Rub it on any problem areas — nose, forehead, that sort of thing.

3. That's it! We told you it was laughably easy!

Recipe #7:
Easy DIY Blackhead Remover

Considering they're such small dots on your face, blackheads can get a surprising number of people riled up and shaking their bottles of exfoliating cream in frustration. Blackheads, which are caused by clogged pores, can really ruin someone's day, next to an otherwise immaculate complexion. This laughably easy recipe helps to tighten the pores, squeeze out excess sebum and prevent more of these little blighters from forming.

Ingredients:

- 1/2 fresh lemon
- 1/2 tsp raw honey
- 1/4 tsp sugar (any sugar will do, but if possible stick to standard cane sugar)

Recipe #8:
Moisturizing Hair and Scalp Treatment

Over time, your hair and scalp can dry out and become brittle. You can even develop dandruff, especially if you regularly shampoo, dye or use a lot of products in your hair. This wonderful-smelling recipe will help to cleanse your hair follicles and scalp of product build-up and sebum. It will also hydrate your hair and even help to stimulate hair growth. We think that after using it once, you'll want to add it to your regular beauty routine!

Ingredients:

- 4 tbsp coconut oil
- 2 drops tea tree essential oil
- 3 drops rosemary essential oil
- 2 tbsp lemon juice
- 1 tbsp grapefruit juice

Equipment:

- Small bowl
- Natural bristle brush
- Paint brush or basting brush to apply mixture

Instructions:

1. Squeeze the fresh citrus juice, and mix the ingredients together in a small bowl.

2. Brush hair thoroughly with natural bristle brush to increase circulation and remove dry skin.

3. Center-part hair and begin applying mixture with application brush, section by section.

4. Massage scalp thoroughly for a few minutes, and leave mixture on for 20 minutes. Rinse or wash hair afterward.

Recipe #9:
Meyer Lemon Salt Scrub

After you try this amazing-smelling salt scrub for the first time, you'll quickly become the envy of your friends and coworkers for your glowing skin and blissfully radiant complexion. Meyer lemon, sea salt, freshly chopped thyme and almond oil combine in this recipe to make one seriously effective skin treatment.

Ingredients:

- 1 cup sea salt
- 1/2 cup organic almond oil
- Zest of 1 Meyer lemon
- 2 tsp fresh thyme, leaves stripped from stem

Equipment:

- Sterilized glass jar or container with lid

Instructions:

1. Combine the sea salt, lemon zest and fresh thyme in a clean, sterilized glass jar or container with a tight-fitting lid.

2. Pour the almond oil over the rest of the ingredients and tightly screw on the lid.

3. Each time you want to use the scrub, simply use a spoon to combine the ingredients together, scoop some out and use it as a scrub in the shower.

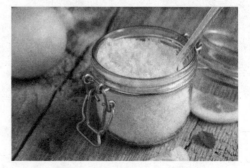

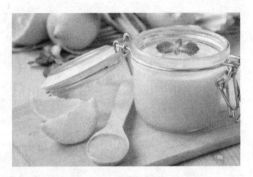

Recipe #10:
Lemon Cream Body Butter

One of the best ways to treat tired, dry skin is with a healthy dose of body butter. While conventional body butters may achieve this, they're also expensive and can introduce harmful chemicals into your body through your skin (which, many people are surprised to learn, is highly absorbent).

This luxurious body butter, on the other hand, is composed of healthy, natural ingredients that won't break the bank and will get your skin back into ship shape in no time. If you have sensitive skin, be aware that the citrus oils in this recipe can increase sensitivity to the sun.

Ingredients:

- 6 tbsp coconut oil
- 1/4 cup cacao butter
- 1 tbsp vitamin E oil
- 5 drops lemon essential oil

Equipment:

- Saucepan and bowl to make a double boiler
- Glass jar for storage

Instructions:

1. Melt the coconut oil and butter together in a double boiler.

2. Remove from heat and cool for a few minutes, then add the vitamin E oil and lemon essential oil.

3. Allow to cool completely, then scoop into a jar for storage. Enjoy the luxurious, rich texture!

Recipe #11:
Lemon Rosemary Lip Balm

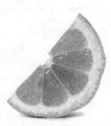

Have you ever accidentally licked your lips after putting on lip balm and worried about the ingredients being introduced into your body? Well, with this homemade lip balm, you don't have to worry! With the all-natural ingredients and delicious flavor and aroma, it makes a healthy replacement for your usual store-bought balm. It even provides sun protection for your lips with the added oils!

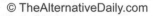

Ingredients:

- 1/2 cup almond oil
- 3 tbsp beeswax
- 1 tsp vitamin E oil
- 15 drops lemon essential oil
- 15 drops rosemary essential oil
- 15 drops raspberry seed oil
- 15 drops carrot seed oil

Equipment:

- Saucepan and bowl to make a double boiler
- Lip balm tube or small glass jar for storage

Instructions:

1. In a double boiler, combine the almond oil and beeswax until melted.

2. Once melted, remove the bowl from heat and add in vitamin E, raspberry seed, carrot seed, lemon and rosemary essential oils.

3. Mix together and pour into lip balm tubes or small jars. Let sit until cool and solidified.

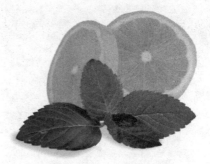

Recipe #12:
Cooling Peppermint Foot Scrub

Been on your feet all day at work, trained for that upcoming half marathon or spent the whole day exploring the streets of an exotic city on foot? Whatever reason you had for spending so much time on your feet, chances are they're feeling hot, swollen and just a little bit unloved.

The peppermint in this foot scrub provides a glorious cooling sensation for your overworked feet, while the lemon helps to freshen your skin and keep your feet looking their best.

Ingredients:

- 1 cup coarse sea salt
- 1/2 cup sweet almond oil
- 2 tsp lemon zest
- 6 drops peppermint essential oil

Equipment:

- Small glass bowl
- Clean jar with lid

Instructions:

1. Combine all the ingredients in a small glass bowl, and then transfer to a clean jar with a lid.

2. When you're ready to use it, use your hands to firmly massage the scrub into your feet. Pay particular attention to your heels and any other areas that seem a little bit worse for wear.

3. Leave on for 5 to 10 minutes, then rinse off with warm water. Immediately rub some coconut oil or more of the almond oil onto your feet to lock in the moisture.

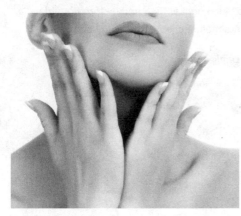

Recipe #13:
Lemon Rosemary Detox Scrub

This recipe not only leaves skin looking smooth and bright, but also helps excrete toxins and fight bloating. The olive oil and salt combination is exfoliating, moisturizing and nourishing, while the lemon and rosemary are invigorating and detoxifying.

Ingredients:

- 1 1/2 cups Epsom salt
- 4 tbsp of olive oil
- Juice of 1-2 lemons
- Zest of one lemon
- 2 sprigs of fresh rosemary

Equipment:

- Tall glass jar
- Large mixing bowl

Instructions:

1. Add salt to a large bowl and mix in the juice of two lemons with the zest of one lemon. Stir to combine.

2. Add olive oil and mix thoroughly. Let it sit while you finely chop your rosemary leaves.

3. Combine all ingredients together into a tall glass jar.

4. Store in the refrigerator and mix or shake before use.

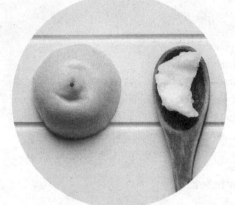

Equipment:

- Spray bottle

Instructions:

1. Combine all ingredients in spray bottle and shake to mix.

2. Apply to damp hair and scrunch gently to encourage waves.

Recipe #15:
Quick and Easy Acne Treatment

You may have left your teen years behind, but you're still not immune to the odd bout of acne. Even worse than a big ol' zit is the scar it can sometimes leave behind. This simple recipe is an effective, natural treatment for acne and scars. It works like a charm but is much gentler than harsh store-bought or prescription chemical formulations.

Ingredients:

- Juice of 1/4 lemon
- 1 tsp cinnamon

Equipment:

- Cotton balls
- Small bowl

Recipe #14:
Beach Hair Spray

Some people put a whole lot of time and money into getting that glorious, textured, wavy hair that comes from a day spent at the seaside. Conveniently, this time we've brought the beach to you, with this easy-to-make and even easier-to-use recipe. Not only will your hair look amazing and get a sun-kissed lightening effect, it'll smell great too!

Ingredients:

- 1 cup warm water
- 1 tbsp sea salt
- Juice of 1/2 lemon
- 2 tsp coconut oil

Instructions:

1. Mix the lemon juice and cinnamon together in a small bowl.

2. Apply the paste to acne-affected areas.

3. Let sit for 15 minutes, then rinse with warm water. Repeat daily as needed.

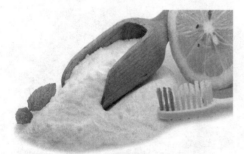

Recipe #16:
Lemon Teeth-Whitening Treatment

Lemon can help to whiten your teeth in a number of ways. It's a great source of vitamin C, an antioxidant that acts as a bleaching agent to clear away yellow discoloration on the enamel of your teeth. Lemon also has anti-bacterial properties to prevent the development of teeth-staining bacteria and discourage oral diseases. Finally, it contains citric acid, which stimulates saliva production that in turn cleanses your mouth.

This teeth-whitening recipe harnesses the oral power of the lemon while avoiding all of the expenses and toxins associated with conventional teeth whitening treatments. It'll leave you with a brighter, whiter smile in no time.

Ingredients:

- Juice of 1/4 lemon
- 1 tbsp baking soda

Equipment:

- Small bowl
- Toothbrush

Instructions:

1. Mix together the freshly squeezed lemon juice and baking soda in a small bowl.

2. Scoop up the mixture with your toothbrush and brush your teeth gently. Leave on for a minute or two, then rinse.

3. Repeat the treatment weekly for beautiful white teeth.

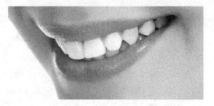

Recipe #17:
Lemon Hair Gel

If you spend hours battling your frizz and trying to get it to resemble something even remotely close to fashionable, this homemade lemon hair gel recipe is just the ticket. It sidesteps all the nasty toxins found in your average tub of hair gel, and it's amazingly easy to make. Your hair, and your fashion sense, will thank you for it!

Ingredients:

- 1 tbsp gelatin
- 1 cup water
- 2 tbsp lemon juice
- 1-2 tsp coconut oil, in liquid form (optional)
- 4 tbsp aloe vera gel (optional)

Equipment:

- Blender
- Airtight jar for storage

Instructions:

1. In a saucepan over medium heat, mix water with gelatin until it has completely dissolved.

2. Remove from heat and mix in lemon juice. Let cool until the mixture has formed into a gel.

3. For an optional conditioning addition to the hair gel, mix in coconut oil and aloe vera before the gel completely sets. Place everything in a blender and blend on low until it becomes a creamy consistency.

4. Store in an airtight jar, and scoop a tablespoon out every time you want to tame the frizz.

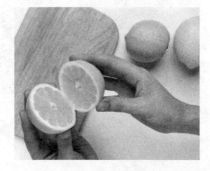

Lemons Throughout the Home

Household cleaners are some of the worst offenders when it comes to daily chemical exposure. Some of the toxins found in common household cleaners include:

- Phthalate: disrupts the endocrine system, has also been shown to significantly lower sperm count in men.

- Perchloroethylene: neurotoxin and possible carcinogen. Immediate symptoms include dizziness and loss of coordination.

- Triclosan: possible endocrine disruptor, possible carcinogen and aggressive antibacterial agent which promotes the growth of harmful, resistant bacterial strains.

- 2-Butoxyethanol: high levels of this compound can cause narcosis, pulmonary edema and severe liver and kidney damage.

- Ammonia: this is a powerful irritant. Long-term exposure promotes the development of chronic bronchitis and asthma.

You get the idea. Store-bought cleaners are almost always bad for your health and can put your livelihood at risk. At worst, they can promote the development of life-threatening diseases and conditions. Rather than searching for products that claim to be cleaner or "toxin-free," why not turn to the simplest, most effective option? The humble lemon!

Utilizing the power of fresh lemon juice can provide all the benefits of a conventional household cleaner, leave your home smelling fresh, and support (rather than degrade) your health in the process. That's what they call a win-win!

Try these easy recipes to get your home lemony-fresh, without the toxins.

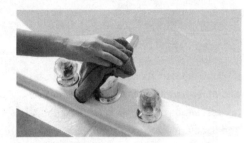

Recipe #18: Soap Scum Remover

Even for the most vigilant cleaner, soap scum can be a real pain in the butt to get the better of. It builds up quickly, and can make even the most lavish bathroom look dirty and unappealing. Use the cleaning power of the lemon with this easy solution to quickly and efficiently remove soap scum.

Ingredients:

- 1 lemon
- Warm water

Equipment:

- Scrub brush

Instructions:

1. Cut lemon in half.

2. Rub the juicy side of the lemon over areas affected by soap scum. Let sit a few minutes.

3. Scrub gently with brush and rinse with warm water. Repeat as needed.

The Alternative Daily

Recipe #19:
Cutting Board Disinfectant

If you're worried about buildup of bacteria and other harmful pathogens on your cutting boards, we have just the thing. This natural, non-toxic application will disinfect even the dirtiest of cutting boards —it's particularly effective on those made of wood or bamboo.

Ingredients:

- 1 lemon
- 1 tbsp sea salt
- Warm water

Instructions:

1. Cut lemon in half and sprinkle with sea salt.
2. Rub the lemon on the cutting board, letting the juice seep in for a few minutes.
3. Rinse well and enjoy your clean cutting board!

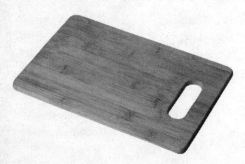

Recipe #20:
Lemon Copper Polisher

Over time, your treasured copper bowls and kitchen utensils can become tarnished and look less than ideal. Rather than making a trip down to the store to buy some toxic, overpriced polishing agent, why not try this amazingly simple solution instead? It works just as well, and it doesn't require you to come into contact with harmful toxins.

Ingredients:

- 1 whole lemon, cut in half
- 1 tsp coarse sea salt

Instructions:

1. Take a lemon half, dip it in the coarse sea salt, and rub it across the copper surface.
2. After you've covered the full surface of the copper item, leave for 10 minutes.
3. Buff off with a clean cloth.

Hint: while this is a tried and true solution, it's always best to test your lemon rub on a small, unnoticeable area first.

Recipe #21:
No-Bleach Laundry Whitener

Bleach has got to be one of the most harmful chemicals we keep around the house. In many homes it provides the backbone for cleaning mold and mildew from bathrooms and whitening clothes. However, its high chlorine content makes it highly corrosive and capable of irritating your eyes, skin, lungs and respiratory tract. How willing are you to harm your health for the sake of a whiter t-shirt?

Luckily, there's an easier, healthier solution — and once again, it's surprisingly simple! Try this lemon application for an alternative, all-natural laundry whitener.

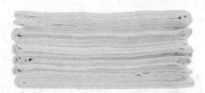

Ingredients:

- 1 lemon
- Hot water

Equipment:

- Large bucket or basin

Instructions:

1. Mix the juice of the lemon with hot water in a large basin.

2. Add clothing and let soak for 1 to 2 hours.

3. Wring out clothing and allow it to dry in the sun. The combination of the lemon and sunlight amazingly brightens whites.

4. Wash as usual, if desired.

Recipe #22:
All-Purpose Cleaning Solution

Vinegar is quickly becoming a popular natural alternative to conventional household cleaners due to its strong antibacterial and anti-fungal properties. Add the antimicrobial powers and amazing smell of lemon, and you've got yourself a highly effective homemade cleaner and gentle disinfectant. You can use this on essentially any surface in your house.

Ingredients:

- 1/2 cup white vinegar
- Juice of 1 lemon
- 2 cups water

The Alternative Daily

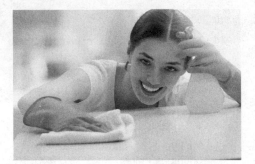

Equipment:

- Glass bottle with spray topper

Instructions:

1. Combine ingredients in spray bottle and shake to mix.

2. Simply spray on surface, allow it to sit for a minute, then wipe clean.

Recipe #23:
Lemon Stain Remover

We've all been there —you just bought a nice white shirt, and you're giving it a whirl at a dinner party at a friend's house. Then, inevitably, you spill a bit of fruit salad, wine or meat juice smack bang in the middle of that pristine whiteness. You bitterly regret ever making the decision to buy something so obviously stain-attracting!

But don't despair, there's a natural, easy treatment for those stains, and it doesn't involve using those foul-smelling, toxic stain removers you get in the store. Check out this recipe for all your stain removing needs.

Ingredients:

- Juice from 1 lemon
- Water (as needed)
- Baking soda (as needed)

Equipment:

- Bucket or laundry tub

Instructions:

1. After a strain, cut a lemon in half and squeeze the juice directly into a bucket or laundry sink as soon as possible.

2. Place the stained clothing item in the receptacle, fill with water, and leave for at least 1 hour.

3. If the stain persists, dampen the area and make a paste out of equal parts baking soda and water. Scrub gently.

4. After treating, either rinse the garment with warm water or throw it straight into the washing machine.

Recipe #24:
Grout Cleaner

Tiles in the kitchen or bathroom look great and are generally easy to clean, but the grouting between those tiles is a different matter altogether. Because most grout is light in color and slightly porous, it can quickly and easily become discolored and loaded with dirt, grime and bacteria. If this is the case in your home, try this lemon-based cleaner for natural brightening and scrubbing power.

Ingredients:

- Juice of 1 lemon
- 2 tsp baking soda

Equipment:

- Small bowl
- Old toothbrush

Instructions:

1. Mix the lemon juice and baking soda together to form a paste.
2. Apply to grout with toothbrush and let sit for a few minutes.
3. Give it a good scrub, and rinse well.

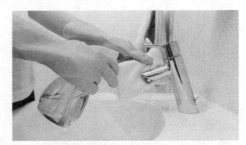

Recipe #25:
Kitchen and Bathroom Sink Cleaner

Over time, sinks in the bathroom or kitchen start to develop a filmy appearance, which looks unsightly and can harbor bacteria and mold. This simple lemon-based cleaner works wonders and will have your metal and ceramic sinks looking shiny and new in no time!

Ingredients:

- Juice of 1 lemon
- 3 tbsp sea salt

Equipment:

- Small bowl
- Scrubbing cloth

Instructions:

1. Mix the lemon juice and salt together in a small bowl to form a scrubbing paste.
2. Use a cloth to work it into surfaces and remove tough dirt. Rinse well.

Recipe #26:
Lemon Garbage Disposal Freshener

Garbage disposals are highly convenient, but over time they can harbor small chunks of food and bacteria, which creates a strong, unpleasant stench. Rather than turning to some chemical-ridden cleaner from your supermarket, why not use this natural, easy, cost-free solution instead?

Ingredients:

- Zest from 1/4 to 1/2 lemon

Equipment:

- Small bowl
- Scrubbing cloth

Instructions:

1. Rather than throwing a lemon away after you use the juice, cut off a quarter to a half of the skin (zest) and place in your garbage disposal.

2. Turn on the faucet and switch on your garbage disposal for an instant lemon scent, which kills any smelly bacteria and keeps your disposal smelling lemon-fresh for days.

Hint: Be sure to avoid putting large chunks of lemon in the disposal, as they can clog or damage the blades.

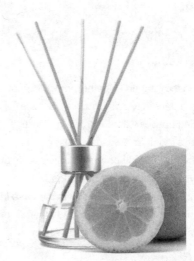

Recipe #27:
Natural Air Freshener

Store-bought air fresheners are highly toxic, and can seriously damage your health. Many contain phthalates (often masked as "fragrance" or "parfum" in the ingredients), which are linked to a range of health conditions. They also commonly contain 1,4-dichlorobenzene, which is a known carcinogen associated with kidney and testicular cancer, and results in lung conditions (such as asthma). And that's just the tip of the iceberg — a 2007 study of 74 different air fresheners available on the market found more than 350 different chemicals and allergens in many of these products. That's a whole lot of toxic!

Your best course of action is to avoid conventional air fresheners altogether — it's just not worth it! However, this leaves you with a bit of a dilemma: how do you keep your home smelling fresh and clean without the aid of toxic products you've relied on in the past? We have the answer! It smells amazing and it's super duper easy.

Ingredients:

- 4 cups water
- Peel from 1 lemon
- 3 cinnamon sticks
- 1 tsp whole cloves
- Splash of vanilla extract, or whole vanilla bean

Equipment:

- Saucepan

Instructions:

1. Place all ingredients in a saucepan.
2. Turn on the heat until the mixture simmers.
3. Keep it going on low for 1-2 hours. This works great for parties and gatherings, or when you just want your home to feel extra pleasant!

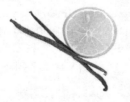

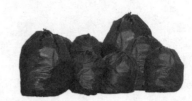

Recipe #28: Garbage Deodorizer

Have you ever bought scented bin liners to keep the garbage and recycling area fresh? Unfortunately, these scented bags contain phthalates and parabens, which are toxic chemicals used to make those resilient scents. Try this chemical-free solution instead.

Ingredients:

- 2 lemons
- 2 oranges

Equipment:

- Lemon zester

Instructions:

1. Use the zester to remove the peels of the lemons and oranges. Doesn't that smell amazing?
2. Put a handful of zest at the bottom of each bin you would like to keep fresh. The essential oils from the citrus fruits will disinfect and deodorize the bins while repelling pests.
3. Repeat every few weeks as needed.

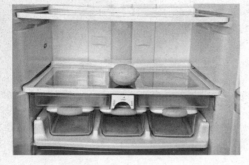

Recipe #29:
Freshen the Refrigerator

Did you know that lemon is an amazing natural deodorizer and disinfectant? Unleash fresh lemon on your refrigerator and get rid of any unpleasant odors fast.

Ingredients:

- 1/2 fresh lemon

Equipment:

- Small bowl
- Cotton balls

Instructions:

1. Squeeze fresh lemon juice into a small bowl.

2. Dab a few cotton balls in lemon juice, and place them around the refrigerator.

3. Leave the cotton balls in place for several hours, then discard.

Recipe #30:
Microwave Cleaner

You've told your kids to cover their plates and bowls of food in the microwave, but the stains covering the inside suggest that, unsurprisingly, they haven't been following orders. Rather than spending hours trying to scrape away all that hardened grime, try this natural lemony solution instead.

Ingredients:

- 1 lemon
- Water

Equipment:

- Glass bowl

Instructions:

1. Cut the lemon in half and squeeze the juice into the bowl.

2. Fill the bowl with water, then place the squeezed lemon halves inside.

3. Place the bowl in the microwave.

4. Run the microwave on high for about 3 minutes to bring the mixture to a boil. Allow the bowl to sit in the microwave for at least 15 minutes to steam treat cooked-on messes.

5. Afterward, the microwave will be much easier to clean. Simply wipe down and enjoy the fresh scent.

Recipe #31:
Natural Furniture Polish

Conventional furniture polishes are often highly poisonous in nature. They contain hydrocarbons that lead to toxic effects when swallowed, inhaled or sprayed into the eyes. What's more, regular furniture polish use can lead to chronic exposure to formaldehyde, a carcinogen that can accumulate in human fat tissue over time. Oh, did we mention that it's also nasty for the environment?

Take the health of your family and the environment back into your own hands with this simple, natural furniture polish. It uses unrefined oils to get your furniture gleaming and polished, and the real lemon juice imparts an amazing fresh scent. Hooray for real things!

Ingredients:

- 1/2 cup freshly squeezed lemon juice
- 1/2 cup olive oil
- Peels from one lemon

Equipment:

- Small glass jar for storage

Instructions:

1. Mix the ingredients together in the glass jar.

2. Seal and allow to sit for one week.

3. Strain the peels, then it's ready to use!

4. Apply a small amount to furniture with a clean cloth. Allow to sit for 15-30 minutes, then wipe down for a gorgeous shine.

Recipe #32:
Non-Toxic Lemon Window Cleaner

Many window cleaners contain nerve-damaging butyl cellosolve, and many others are loaded with ammonia, which can irritate and damage airways. If some window cleaners are accidentally mixed with chlorine-containing cleaners, they can release toxic chloramine gas.

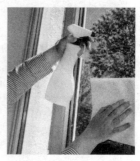

While we recognize that you need to keep those windows fingerprint-free and clean enough to see through (especially when you have guests over!), conventional window cleaners clearly aren't worth the risk. This tried and true recipe uses the streak-free cleaning power of both lemons and white vinegar to make an effective, natural alternative.

Ingredients:

- 4 cups water
- 1/2 cup white vinegar
- 1/2 cup freshly squeezed lemon juice

Equipment:

- Glass bottle with spray topper

Instructions:

1. Combine all ingredients in spray bottle.
2. Seal and shake to combine.
3. Use just like regular window-washing fluid! Just spray down and wipe clean.

Recipe #33:
Handy Grease Remover

Getting your hands covered in grease is common enough around the house, particularly if you're doing renovations to furniture, working with vehicles or motorized items (like that darn broken lawn mower), or shredding the meat from a roast chicken. This grease creates a problem — the only way you can properly remove it from your hands is by using harsh chemical soaps that strip the natural oils from your skin, leaving them dry and sore.

This natural lemon solution lets you sidestep the chemicals yet still remove the grease from your hands quickly and efficiently. Plus, they'll smell great afterwards!

Ingredients:

- 1/2 a lemon
- Bowl of water

Instructions:

1. Rub lemon juice on your hands, and then dip them in the bowl of water.
2. Rub your hands together under the water until all the lemon and grease disappears from your hands.
3. You may need to rinse your wrists off with warm water afterwards, to remove any grease that floated to the water surface during your scrubbing.

Recipe #34:
Non-Toxic Insect Repellent

Bugs hate the smell of fresh lemon. Try these simple solutions to keep insects out of your home without toxic chemicals.

Ingredients:

- 5 lemons

Equipment:

- Lemon zester
- Spray bottle
- Mop and bucket

Instructions:

1. Use the zester to remove the rind of the lemons and save the zest.

2. Juice all of the lemons and set the juice aside.

3. Mix 1/5 of the juice with equal parts water and put in a spray bottle. Use this mixture to spray thresholds and windowsills where bugs are known to enter.

4. Sprinkle some of the lemon zest around the outdoor entrances and sills.

5. Use the rest of the lemon zest and juice to make a floor-washing solution. Mix the zest and juice in a bucket with 1/2 gallon of water. Use this to mop the floors and your home will be ultra lemony-fresh and insect-free!

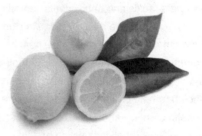

Lemon Recipes for Health and Well-Being

As we already suggested in the earlier sections of this book, lemons are absolutely brimming with beneficial vitamins and nutrients. They contain a group of antioxidants called flavonoids, hard working compounds which fight off cancer and even help to slow the process of aging. They also contain more vitamins than your average multivitamin supplement, with plenty of vitamin C, vitamin B6, vitamin E, folate, niacin, thiamin and riboflavin.

And it doesn't stop there. Lacking in certain essential minerals? Lemons can help with that too! They have high concentrations of copper, calcium, iron, magnesium, potassium, zinc and phosphorus. Not bad for a simple yellow fruit, right?

Due to their potent collection of vitamins, minerals, acids and antioxidants, lemons continue to receive a lot of scientific study from the medical and alternative health communities. To name but a few of their many health benefits, lemons have been shown to help prevent diabetes, alleviate constipation, lower elevated blood pressure, reduce fever, quell indigestion and, of course, fight cancer.

The following recipes harness the knowledge gained from this scientific research, along with extensive anecdotal evidence, to provide you with solutions to many everyday health problems and ailments. They make a great addition to a nutritious diet and preventative wellness routine, and range from simple tonics to complex medicinal preparations. You're sure to find one to fit every need.

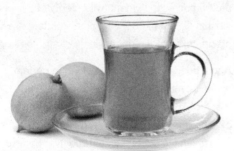

Recipe #35:
Simple Morning Tonic

This super simple morning tonic is so magically health supporting that it has attained something of a cult following in the alternative health world. Add it to your morning routine and you'll be amazed with the benefits it provides, like boosting immunity and cleansing toxins. It's also an early-morning, caffeine-free pick-me-up.

Ingredients:
- Organic lemons
- Filtered water

Equipment:
- Citrus squeezer, if desired

Instructions:
1. Every morning before you consume anything else, drink a glass of room-temperature water with lemon juice. Simply squeeze 1/2 of a fresh lemon into the water, and enjoy.

Hint: Freeze lemon juice into an ice cube tray so you always have some on hand.

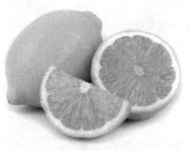

Recipe #36:
Lemon Ginger Tonic

This is a great daily drink as a preventative immunity-booster, but it really shines when you're coming down with a nasty cold or sore throat. The lemons help to support your immune system and cleanse built-up toxins from your liver. The raw honey soothes a sore throat and is naturally antibacterial. The ginger contains a wide range of anti-inflammatory compounds that support your body and strengthen your system against bacterial, viral or fungal attack.

Drink it cold on a hot day, or sip it warm from a mug on a cold night.

Ingredients:

- 3 cups warm filtered water
- 1/2 cup fresh lemon juice
- 1/4 cup raw honey
- 1 tbsp freshly grated ginger
- Ice cubes (optional)

Equipment:

- Blender (optional)

Instructions:

1. Dissolve the honey in the warm water.

2. Add the rest of the ingredients and pulse the mixture in a blender to combine well. This recipe makes two tall glasses, so enjoy with a friend!

3. If you would rather drink this tonic iced, simply make according to the recipe, then add ice cubes, or let chill in the fridge for a while before drinking.

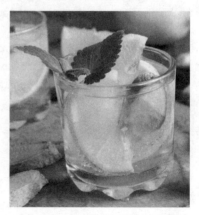

Recipe #37:
Healthy Lemon Sports Drink

Many people like to push their body to the limit, be that at the gym lifting weighty dumbbells and performing intense Tabata workouts, to running long distances or spending a whole day on the slopes carving up powder. Whatever the reason, these activities can strain our bodies, deplete our electrolytes and dehydrate our cells — a situation that needs rectifying ASAP, unless you want a splitting headache or aching joints.

This healthy lemon electrolyte drink does everything your average bottle of Gatorade can do, plus it's actually good for you! It provides plenty of electrolytes to rehydrate the body quickly, and it doesn't introduce synthetic compounds and artificial sugars into your system.

Ingredients:

- Juice from 1 whole lemon
- 1 tsp Himalayan pink salt or unrefined sea salt
- 1 tsp raw honey
- 1/2 tsp organic cinnamon powder

Instructions:

1. Add all the ingredients into your drink bottle, top off with water, and shake thoroughly to mix all the ingredients together.

2. That's it! Your sports drink is ready to roll, however you may need to occasionally shake it to ensure the honey and salt remain suspended in the water.

Recipe #38:
Cayenne Lemonade

Cayenne pepper is well known for its ability to energize the body, improve circulation and lower inflammation in and around the joints. Combine these benefits with the liver-cleansing, cell-hydrating, immunity-boosting lemon and you've got yourself a highly effective, natural energy drink! Forget Red Bull, there's a new kid in town, and this kid doesn't harm your health as it elevates your energy levels and kicks lethargy in the butt. Enjoy warm or cold.

Ingredients:

- 3/4 cup freshly squeezed lemon juice
- 1/2 tsp cayenne pepper
- 1/4 cup raw honey
- 1 cup water

Instructions:

1. Dissolve honey in a little warm (not hot or boiling) water.
2. Add the rest of the ingredients, and top up with the temperature of water that you desire for drinking.

Recipe #39:
Probiotic Kale Lemon Tonic

If your digestion needs a boost or you have reason to believe that your gut microbiome is not what it should be, this probiotic drink is just the thing you need. It combines the nutrients of kale, the probiotic power of raw apple cider vinegar and the immunity-boosting benefits of lemon to get your stomach back on track and get your gut repopulated with beneficial bacteria. It's also a great alkalizer and liver cleanser.

Ingredients:

- 1 cup water
- 1 tbsp raw apple cider vinegar
- Handful organic kale, chopped
- 1 whole lemon, peeled
- 1 tbsp raw honey

Equipment:

- Blender

Instructions:

1. Blend up all ingredients thoroughly.
2. Add more water as needed to adjust consistency, or crushed ice if desired.

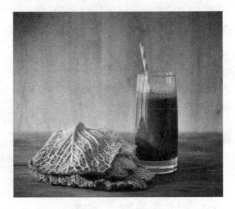

Recipe #40:
Ginger Lemon Jasmine Kombucha

If apple cider vinegar is a little too strong for your taste, kombucha makes a great probiotic alternative. If you don't already make your own, it's super easy to do — just pop down to your local supermarket and buy a bottle of raw, unfiltered kombucha with the SCOBY/mother. Once home, boil some green or black tea and add some sugar. Add some of the kombucha mix and the mother once the tea mixture has cooled. This way, you'll have an endless supply of health-giving kombucha at your fingertips, and you can make as much of this delicious tonic as you could possibly desire!

This recipe adds some tasty, aromatic ingredients to your regular brew of kombucha to spice things up a little and tantalize your tastebuds.

Ingredients:

- 4-6 cups boiling water
- 5 organic jasmine tea bags
- 3/4 cups sugar
- Kombucha SCOBY
- 1/2 cup of previous batch of kombucha
- 1/2 lb fresh ginger root
- 2 lemons

Equipment:

- 3 16-oz jars or bottles for kombucha storage

Instructions:

1. Place boiling water, tea bags and sugar in a large jar. Mix well and leave to cool.

2. Once the tea has cooled, add your SCOBY and cover the jar with fabric and an elastic band. Ferment for 14 days.

3. After this period, make ginger juice by chopping the ginger root into chunks and putting it in the blender for 3-4 minutes. Strain out the pulp. Store extra in ice cube trays for future use.

4. Juice the lemons and set aside.

5. Prepare 3 16-oz bottles or jars, putting 2 tablespoons ginger juice and 2 tablespoons lemon juice in each. Top up with the jasmine kombucha. Use the SCOBY for the next batch of fresh sweetened tea.

6. Put on the lids and put aside for secondary fermentation for 3 to 5 days. Then place in the fridge. Enjoy chilled!

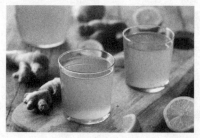

Recipe #41:
Strawberry Kombucha Lemonade

If you're having trouble trying to convince your kids to drink probiotics to keep their good bacteria levels high and protect against illness and infection, mix up this recipe and don't tell them it has kombucha in it. Chances are they'll enjoy the taste so much that they won't ever suspect that it's actually good for them! It's sweet and delicious, yet still low in sugar content.

Ingredients:

- Large jar of prepared kombucha
- 4 organic strawberries
- 1/2 organic lemon

Instructions:

1. When your batch of kombucha has fermented (primary fermentation), slice up strawberries and lemon into thin slices.

2. Add fruit to kombucha, and seal the jar. Allow secondary fermentation to occur for at least 24 hours. The fruit flavors will soak in during this time.

3. Place in the fridge, and enjoy chilled!

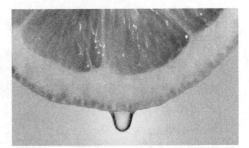

Recipe #42:
Lemon Ginger Turmeric Tea

Tea is a great way to introduce nutrients into the body, soothe the throat and steady the mind. Steeping fresh ingredients in scalding water forces the nutrients to leach out into the water, making them easier for our digestive systems to absorb and put to good work. This tea combines the collective might of three superfood giants — lemon, ginger and turmeric — to make one of the most health-supporting teas you'll ever set your lips to!

Use it when you feel a cold or flu coming on, or drink every day to keep your body happy and healthy.

The Alternative Daily

Ingredients:

- 1 1/2 cups filtered drinking water
- 1 tsp fresh grated turmeric root
- 1 tsp fresh grated ginger root
- Juice of half a lemon
- 1/4 tsp fresh ground black pepper
- 1 tsp raw honey (optional)

Instructions:

1. Add the turmeric, ginger and water to a saucepan over medium heat. Simmer for 5-10 minutes, but do not let the mixture come to a boil.

2. Remove from heat and strain the liquid into a mug.

3. After the mixture has cooled to the point where you can dip a finger in without burning it, mix in the lemon, honey and ground black pepper (the pepper allows your body to break down the nutrients in turmeric more efficiently).

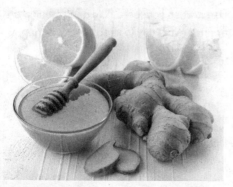

Recipe #43: Fire Cider

With the cold days of winter knocking on your door and the next cold and flu season just around the corner, this recipe is a must-have. It will boost immune systems, keep germs at bay, alleviate the symptoms of colds and flus and provide vital nutrition and fuel for the body during those cold winter months. An especially vital concoction if you have kids around the house, and all the germs and bacteria that come inside with them!

Ingredients:

- 1/2 cup peeled and shredded/diced ginger root
- 1/2 cup peeled and shredded/diced horseradish root
- 1/2 cup peeled and diced turmeric root (or 1/4 cup additional ginger and 1/4 cup additional horseradish)
- 1/2 cup white onion, chopped
- 1/4 cup minced or crushed garlic cloves
- 2 organic jalapeno peppers, chopped
- Zest and juice from 2 organic lemons
- Raw apple cider vinegar
- Raw organic honey to taste

Equipment:

- Large glass jar
- Wax paper
- Cheesecloth or sieve

Instructions:

1. Add the ginger, horseradish, onion, garlic, jalapeno and lemon juice/zest to a quart-sized jar. Pack them down lightly so that the jar is about 3/4 full. Place heavy roots at the top so that they will weigh down the herbs and jalapenos, which float.

2. Pour a generous amount apple cider vinegar over the roots/vegetables. You want everything to stay under the liquid to prevent spoilage. Keep in mind that some of the roots will expand a little, so top it off well.

3. If you're using a metal lid, line it with wax paper so that the vinegar doesn't corrode it, then put the lid on. Place in a dark, room temperature cabinet for 2-4 weeks (a month is best).

4. When the cider is ready, shake well and then strain the roots/veggies using a cheesecloth or fine mesh sieve. Add honey to taste and store in the fridge.

5. Take 1-2 tablespoons daily as a preventative measure, or 1 tablespoon every three hours if cold and flu symptoms are present.

Recipe #44:
Cucumber Lemon Mint Detox Water

Cucumber is an amazingly hydrating fruit, helping to give your cells the water they need to do their thing and flush out any toxins hanging around in your system. When combined with mint and lemon, you've got yourself a mighty refreshing, delicious summertime drink. Enjoy it over ice on a hot day!

Ingredients:

- 12 cups of cool filtered water
- 3 organic lemons
- 1 small organic cucumber
- 15 organic mint leaves

Equipment:

- Large pitcher

Instructions:

1. Wash the lemons, cucumber and mint thoroughly.

2. Slice the lemons and cucumber thinly.

3. Add all ingredients to pitcher and cover with water.

4. Let chill in the refrigerator for a few hours or overnight. Enjoy over ice in a tall glass.

The Alternative Daily

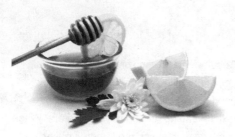

Recipe #45:
Sore Throat Tea

Alright, so you weren't quite quick enough to jump on the preventative health tonic band wagon before that nasty cold hit, but it's okay — we've got a recipe to help with that, too. Lemon is one of the best natural remedies for a sore throat, as it supports the immune system with its high levels of vitamin C. It also helps to kill off the troublesome bacteria causing that niggle in your throat in the first place. And while lemon works its wonders, we've thrown in some delicious raw honey to soothe your throat and help lemon in its antibacterial endeavors.

Ingredients:

- 1 tbsp lemon juice, freshly squeezed
- 2 tbsp raw honey
- Hot water

Instructions:

1. Boil water but allow to cool to drinkable temperature before using. This will protect the enzymes in the raw honey.

2. Pour water into a mug and add honey and lemon juice. Stir well, and sip slowly to soothe a sore throat.

Recipe #46:
Lemon Turmeric Cleansing Smoothie

Smoothies are an excellent way to get a wide range of nutrients in one simple, delicious, easy-to-make meal. This particular smoothie is packed with nutrient-rich, antioxidant-infused, anti-inflammatory ingredients. Use it as a daily morning energy-booster, or perhaps as a hangover cure the morning after having a few too many glasses of wine with friends.

Ingredients:

- 2 cups kale
- 2 cups coconut milk
- 2 cups fresh pineapple
- 1 cup fresh mango
- Juice of 1/2 lemon
- 1 tbsp fresh ginger root
- 1/2 tsp ground turmeric powder

Equipment:

- Blender

Instructions:

1. Place kale and coconut milk in the blender and blend until smooth.

2. Add the remaining ingredients, and blend well.

Hint: If you prefer to enjoy your smoothie cold, place fruits in the freezer before making.

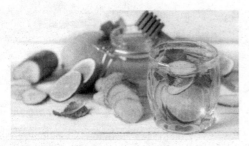

Recipe #47:
Lemon Watermelon Weight-Loss Water

You've probably heard some of the rumors by now about how lemon can help with weight loss, and extensive anecdotal evidence seems to back up this claim. Lemon's ability to rapidly hydrate your cells makes your body feel fuller, so there's less of an urge to overeat.

The ingredients in this water blend are amazingly delicious, but the real power comes in its ability to provide hydration and essential vitamins and minerals for nutrient-starved cells. You'll enjoy it equally over ice on a warm summer day, or as a morning revitalizer on a cold winter morning.

Ingredients:

- 1 sliced organic cucumber
- 1 sliced organic lemon
- 1 tbsp grated organic ginger
- 1/2 cup organic mint leaves
- 6 glasses filtered or mineral water

Equipment:

- Large pitcher or mason jar

Instructions:

1. In your large glass pitcher or mason jar, throw in your cucumber, lemon, ginger and mint leaves.

2. Add the filtered water or mineral water to the pitcher or jar, so that all ingredients are fully immersed in the water.

3. Leave the mixture in the fridge overnight, and then drink a glass of it every morning before breakfast.

Recipe #48:
Lemon Cayenne Slimming Drink

Yes, the previous recipe is delicious and a winner with the whole family, but in case you do get tired of it, this recipe also packs one heck of a punch to unwanted pounds! Cayenne curbs the appetite and speeds up the metabolism, while the maple syrup adds a rich sweetness to the drink and simultaneously improves digestion — all key elements of effective weight loss. Note that the cayenne can give this drink a bit of a kick, so be prepared!

Ingredients:

- 2 tbsp fresh lemon juice
- 2 tsp maple syrup (make sure it's the real deal, not an artificial imposter)
- 1/2 tsp cayenne pepper
- 8 oz filtered water

Instructions:

1. Pour the water into a glass, allowing plenty of extra room for the additional ingredients.

2. Add in the lemon juice, maple syrup and cayenne pepper. Stir well until thoroughly mixed.

3. Drink on a regular basis, particularly before meals, to start working towards that body you've been aiming for.

Recipe #49:
Natural Hangover Remedy

If you over-indulged and you're suffering the day after, try this easy curative drink. The combination of tea and lemon is a sure energizer and detoxifier. This mix helps with other types of headaches too!

Ingredients:

- 1 fresh lemon

Equipment:

- Citrus juicer
- 1 teabag (black or green)
- Kettle

Instructions:

1. Set the kettle to boil. While that is working, juice the lemon.

2. Steep the tea for at least 3 minutes in a covered mug to make a strong brew.

3. Add the lemon juice and enjoy.

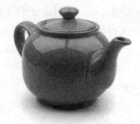

Recipe #50:
Chemical-Free Halitosis Remedy

Got bad breath? We recommend avoiding commercial mouthwash or other treatments that contain artificial colors, flavors or alcohol, which can leave your mucus membranes dried out. This natural alternative encourages balanced bacteria and clean, fresh breath with wholesome ingredients.

Ingredients:

- Juice of 1 lemon
- 1/2 cup pure aloe vera juice or gel (inner leaf)
- 2 tablespoons freshly chopped parsley
- 1/2 cup chopped cucumber
- 5 drops peppermint essential oil, or fresh mint leaves (optional)
- Water

Equipment:

- Blender

Instructions:

1. Place all of the ingredients in the blender.
2. Pulse until smooth.
3. Either drink this green juice daily, or keep a bottle of it in the fridge and rinse your mouth out thoroughly twice per day.

Recipe #51:
Lemon Mood-Booster

If you're having an uninspiring day, try this quick pick-me-up using the bright aroma of lemons.

Ingredients:

- 1/2 fresh lemon
- 1/2 fresh grapefruit
- 1 sprig fresh rosemary, or a handful of basil or mint leaves
- Pot of water

Equipment:

- Blender

Instructions:

1. Slice the lemon and grapefruit into thin slices.
2. Grab your herbs and "bruise" them by squeezing in your hands or mushing them with the bottom of a glass or spoon. This releases the natural oils.
3. Place the citrus and herbs into a small pot of water, and set to a simmer. The amazing aroma will fill your home.
4. Keep checking on the pot once in a while to ensure the water has not gotten too low. This recipe is good to use for 2 to 3 hours.

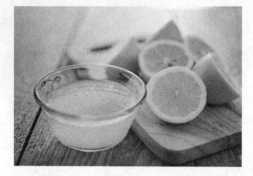

Fun Recipes With Lemons

Okay, enough of the serious stuff. You've smoothed your complexion, strengthened your hair, fortified your body against disease and decay and cleaned your house the healthy way. Now it's time to let loose and experience the taste sensation that is lemon.

The following recipes enlist the strong, tart taste of the lemon and complement it with ingredients that taste great and (believe it or not) are not too shabby for your health either. Recipes range from tasty snacks and hors d'oeuvres for entertaining guests in style, to jazzing up salads or creating delicious natural popsicles.

The opportunities for lemons to spice up your life and tantalize your taste buds are endless... but here's a few to get you started!

Recipe #52:
Sparkling Lemon Punch

Whatever the reason, you don't always want every single drink at a party to be infused with alcohol. Sadly though, many nonalcoholic drinks and punches are boring and tasteless. This beautiful beverage is anything but, providing a delicious, nutritious alcohol-free option at your next shindig. Tasty for adults, and fun and fancy for the kids!

Ingredients:

- Juice of 10 lemons
- Good quality cranberry juice cocktail (minimal sugar)
- 2 bottles club soda or sparkling mineral water
- Fresh mint for garnish

Equipment:

- Large pitcher
- Citrus juicer

Instructions:

1. To start, juice the lemons with the citrus juicer.

2. Mix the lemon juice, cranberry juice and sparkling water together in a large pitcher. Add ice cubes if desired.

3. Store in the fridge until ready to serve. Garnish with fresh mint leaves. Serve in flutes for a fancy treat!

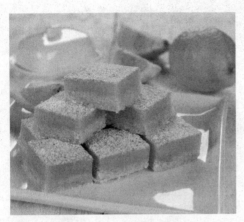

Recipe #53:
Gluten-Free Lemon Squares

This one is a real hit with those who have a niggling sweet tooth, and even those who claim to be indifferent towards desserts! It tastes tart and amazing, and won't raise the hackles on any of the health-conscious eaters in the room.

Ingredients:
Crust:

- 2 cups almond flour
- 6 tbsp sugar
- 3 tbsp gluten-free cornstarch
- 1/4 tsp salt
- 6 tbsp diced cold butter

Filling:

- 2 large eggs
- 1 cup coconut sugar
- 1/3 cup lemon juice
- 2 tbsp gluten-free cornstarch
- Pinch of salt

Equipment:

- Square baking pan

Instructions:

1. Preheat the oven to 350°F. Grease your pan with coconut oil or butter and set aside. Combine the dry crust ingredients in a bowl and whisk together.

2. Add the diced cold butter and work with your fingers until it is a crumbly texture.

3. Put the crust mixture into the greased pan and press flat. Work it a 1/2-inch up the sides of the pan as well.

4. Bake the crust for 8 to 10 minutes, until it looks slightly golden brown.

5. While the crust is baking, whisk the filling ingredients together in another bowl.

6. Pour the filling over the freshly baked crust, and bake for about 15 minutes, until the mixture is set.

7. Refrigerate until you're ready to slice and serve.

67 Ways to Use Lemons Every Day...
Recipes for Health, Beauty and Home!

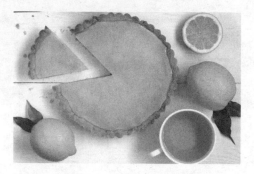

Recipe #54:
Lemon Blender Pie (Gluten-Free)

Sometimes you want to follow up a hearty meal with something delicious and sweet, but just can't find the motivation to spend hours slaving away in the kitchen. With this recipe, there's no excuse not to — it's ridiculously easy to make. It simply requires you to throw everything in a blender, and then transfer ingredients to a pan. Give it a whirl; it'll quickly become a household favorite for simple family meals and guest dinners alike.

Ingredients:

- 3/4 cup white rice flour
- 4 eggs
- 1/3 cup freshly squeezed lemon juice
- 1 cup raw honey
- 1 cup shredded coconut (unsweetened)

- 1 tbsp natural vanilla extract
- 1 1/2 cups hemp milk
- 1/4 cup melted butter
- 1 tsp freshly grated lemon zest

Equipment:

- Pie dish
- Blender

Instructions:

1. Preheat oven to 350°F. Grease pie dish with butter or coconut oil.

2. Put all of the ingredients together in a blender, and blend until smooth. It's that easy!

3. Now just pour the mixture into the pie dish. Bake for about one hour, or until a toothpick comes out clean. The top of the pie should have a golden toasted appearance.

4. Sprinkle with coconut and enjoy with vanilla ice cream or Greek yogurt if desired.

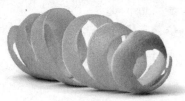

Recipe #55:
Lemon Ricotta Cookies

When it comes to sweet treats, cookies are the undisputed champions of taste and popularity. There must be something about their size that gives them an edge over cakes, pies and pastries... or maybe it's that delicious crunch followed by the tantalizing soft interior that does it. Whatever the reason, we think you'll love this interesting addition to your cookie-baking repertoire.

Ingredients:
Cookies:

- 2 1/2 cups all purpose flour (substitute 1 cup almond flour, 1 cup rice flour and 1/2 cup coconut flour for a gluten-free alternative)
- 1 tsp baking powder
- 1 tsp salt
- 1 stick unsalted butter, softened
- 2 cups coconut sugar (or 1 cup maple syrup)
- 2 eggs
- 1 15-oz container whole milk ricotta cheese
- 3 tbsp lemon juice
- 1 organic lemon, zested

Glaze (optional):

- 1 1/2 cups powdered sugar
- 3 tbsp lemon juice
- Zest from one organic lemon

Equipment:

- Electric mixer

Instructions:

1. Combine the flour, baking powder and salt in a bowl. Set aside.

2. In anther bowl, combine the softened butter and sugar and use an electric mixer to beat the butter and sugar until light and fluffy, approximately 3 minutes.

3. Add the eggs into the butter and sugar mix, beating until incorporated. Add in the ricotta cheese and juice, mixing constantly. Finally, stir in the dry ingredients.

4. Line two baking sheets with parchment paper, then spoon the dough onto the sheets to make cookies of your choosing (2 tablespoons is a good amount per cookie).

5. Bake for 15 minutes, or until golden at the edges. Let cool, and enjoy!

6. The glaze is optional, but if you're feeling really inspired, you can take the cookies to the next level. In a small bowl, mix together powdered

sugar, lemon juice and lemon zest in a small bowl.

7. Once the cookies have cooled (around 20 minutes), spoon approximately half a teaspoon of the glaze onto each cookie and evenly spread across its surface.

8. Place the cookies in the fridge until the glaze has hardened, typically 1-2 hours. Bon appetite!

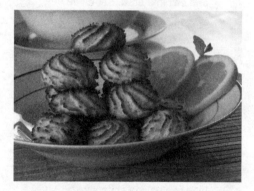

Recipe #56:
Lemon Coconut Macaroons (Gluten-Free)

These little bites are deliciously sweet yet contain very little sugar! Enjoy anytime for a guilt-free treat.

Ingredients:

- 3 large egg whites
- 3 tbsp raw honey
- 2 tbsp freshly squeezed lemon juice (1/2 lemon)
- 1 tsp vanilla extract
- 1/8 tsp salt
- 2 cups unsweetened shredded coconut

Equipment:

- Mixing bowl
- Baking sheet
- Parchment paper
- Hand mixer or whisk

Instructions:

1. Preheat oven to 350°F. Line a baking sheet with parchment paper.

2. In a bowl, whip the egg whites to soft peaks. Add the honey, lemon juice, vanilla and salt and continue whipping until stiff peaks form.

3. Fold in the shredded coconut.

4. Place the mixture in the refrigerator to let it bind.

5. Form into balls and place each one on the baking sheet. The balls should hold together.

6. Bake for 12-15 minutes. Depending on the size of the cookie, a longer baking time might be required. Each recipe makes 15-20 macaroons.

Recipe #57:
Lemon Herb Salmon Burgers

This is a delicious and nutritious main dish that is perfect for summer evenings or to pack along for lunch.

Ingredients:
Salmon Burgers:

- 1 shallot
- 1/2 cup fresh herbs (such as basil and parsley)
- 16 oz wild caught raw salmon, skin removed
- 1 cup cooked quinoa
- 1 egg and 1 egg white
- 1/2 tsp dried herb seasoning mix, such as marjoram, chives, and onion
- 2 tbsp fresh lemon juice
- Salt and pepper to taste

Dressing:

- 2 tbsp minced herbs and shallot (reserved from burgers)
- 1/4 cup avocado oil
- 1/4 cup Greek yogurt
- 2 tbsp water
- 1-2 tbsp fresh lemon juice
- 1/4 tsp salt
- 1 tsp honey

Equipment:

- Food processor

Instructions:

1. Mince the shallot and herbs. Set aside two tablespoons of the shallot/herbs for the dressing.

2. Sauté the remaining shallot and herbs in a little avocado oil over for a few minutes.

3. Pulse the salmon 2-3 times briefly in a food processor until well chopped and a little bit sticky.

4. Stir together with the quinoa, eggs, seasoning, lemon juice, salt, pepper, and the shallots and herbs from step 1. Shape the mixture into four patties.

5. Heat a small drizzle of avocado oil in skillet, then fry the patties, flipping once after 3-4 minutes. The patties should be golden brown on the outside and fully cooked on the inside.

6. Place all the dressing ingredients in a jar and shake until combined (don't forget the reserved shallot and herbs from step 1). Serve over the salmon burgers.

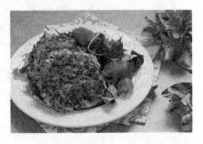

Recipe #58:
Lemony Slaw with Avocado

Spruce up your stock standard slaw with this amazing lemony twist! It's a delicious yet satisfying side dish that goes great with any type of grilled meat or fish. What's more, the critic acid in lemon helps your body to break down and absorb the nutrients locked up in that slaw, and offsets the cabbage nicely. Use organic veggies if you can!

Ingredients:

- 6 cups finely shredded purple and green cabbage
- 1 small bell pepper, chopped
- 1 ripe avocado, diced
- 2 tbsp finely chopped red onion
- 3 tbsp freshly squeezed lemon juice
- 2 tbsp chia seeds
- 1/4 cup chopped cilantro
- 1/4 tsp sea salt
- Freshly ground black pepper, to taste

Instructions:

1. Combine cabbage, pepper, onion, lemon juice, salt and pepper in a large salad bowl, and toss to combine.

2. Add avocado, sprinkle chia seeds and cilantro over top, and toss again gently to combine.

3. Chill up to 2 hours, or serve immediately.

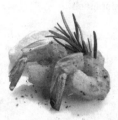

Recipe #59:
Lemon Shrimp

For a break from chicken or beef, try this delicious lemon shrimp recipe. It has plenty of delicious — not to mention nutritious — ingredients. You can have it from pan to table in less than half an hour. It's sure to become a household favorite!

Ingredients:

- 1 1/2 pounds large shrimp, shelled and deveined
- 4 tsp unsalted butter
- 1 tsp finely grated organic lemon zest
- 2 tbsp fresh lemon juice
- 1 tbsp minced fresh dill
- Himalayan pink salt to taste
- Freshly ground black pepper to taste

Instructions:

1. Divide the shrimp evenly between two large plates, and pat dry with a paper towel. Season with salt and pepper.

2. Prepare two large skillets over medium heat. Add a teaspoon of butter to one of the skillets and turn the heat to high. After the butter melts, quickly pour a whole plate of the shrimp into the skillet, spreading them out with a wooden spoon so they cover the surface evenly. Repeat this process with the second skillet.

3. Cook the shrimp until golden brown on the bottom, around 2 minutes. Add another teaspoon of butter to each skillet, and then turn off the heat. Use tongs to turn each shrimp over, and cook for another minute.

4. Add half the lemon zest, lemon juice and dill to each pan and mix around with the wooden spoon to combine.

5. Divide the shrimp up amongst four plates (or two, if you're feeling hungry or you're enjoying a night in with your significant other).

Recipe #60:
Poached Salmon with Lemon Sauce

Not a huge fan of shrimp but still have a hankering for seafood? We've got just the thing! This recipe takes poached salmon, a traditional favorite, and spruces it up with a delightful lemon-mint tzatziki sauce, which will have even the most reserved doubters coming back for second helpings. For the ultimate healthy meal, try to find wild-caught, sustainable salmon instead of the farmed variety.

Ingredients:

- 2 cups water
- 2 cups dry white wine
- 2 bay leaves
- 2 organic lemons, sliced
- 2 sprigs fresh organic parsley
- 1 large salmon fillet, skin on
- 1 cup full-fat yogurt
- 1 English cucumber
- 1 tsp extra virgin olive oil
- 1/2 tsp minced garlic
- 1/4 tsp organic lemon zest
- 1 tbsp finely chopped organic mint leaves
- Himalayan pink salt, to taste
- Fresh ground black pepper, to taste

Equipment:

- Strainer

Instructions:

1. To make the tzatziki, line a strainer with a paper towel and put the strainer over a bowl. Put the yogurt in the strainer and place in the refrigerator to drain for 3 hours.

2. Grate the cucumber, removing seeds if desired. Remove excess water created from the grating.

3. Combine the thickened yogurt and olive oil in a bowl, then stir in the cucumber, lemon juice, lemon zest, garlic and mint. Season with salt and pepper to taste.

4. To make the poached salmon, combine the water, wine, bay leaves, parsley and 1/2 sliced lemon in a large skillet and bring to a simmer.

5. Add the salmon to the skillet, skin side down. If the mix does not cover the salmon, add more water. Place a lid on the skillet and simmer over low heat for around 8 minutes.

6. Place the salmon on a large serving dish, garnish with the remaining sliced lemon and serve alongside the lemon tzatziki sauce you made earlier. Delish!

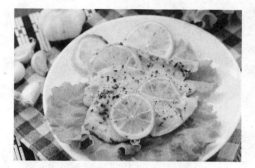

Recipe #61:
Easy Lemon Garlic Chicken

All out of ideas for tasty new dinners or snacks? This recipe is simple and delicious. It can also be made in bulk for use as a protein-rich snack on the go or as an easy salad improver. The chicken also makes a great appetizer, especially with some Greek yogurt and dill dip. Yum!

Ingredients:

- 4 organic chicken breasts, cut into strips
- 4 tsp rice flour, or gluten-free flour mix
- 2 tsp coconut oil
- 1/2 cup organic chicken broth
- 1 tsp minced garlic
- 2 tsp freshly squeezed lemon juice
- 1 tsp butter
- Salt and pepper

Instructions:

1. Flatten chicken slightly. Dust with flour, salt and pepper.

2. Fry in hot oil 5 minutes per side. Remove chicken from pan.

3. To the empty pan add broth, garlic, lemon juice and butter. Cook the sauce for 2 minutes, then pour over chicken.

Recipe #62:
Creamy Lemon Ice Pops

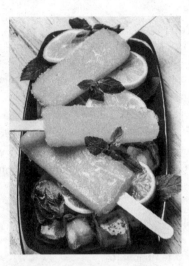

Nothing beats a juicy, chilled ice pop on a hot day — or even on a cold day, for that matter. But while they may provide a treat for your taste buds, they're absolutely loaded with sugar and other ingredients you probably don't even want to think about.

Try this simple recipe instead. It's relatively healthy with a whole lot less sugar than a conventional ice pop. It tastes amazing with the lemon, turning it into a nutritious sorbet. Keep a batch of pre-made lemon ice pops in the freezer for when the kids come calling!

Ingredients:

- 1/2 cup sugar
- 1/4 cup fresh lemon juice
- 2 tbsp grated lemon peel
- Pinch of salt
- 1 1/4 cups buttermilk

Equipment:

- Ice pop molds

Instructions:

1. Whisk sugar, lemon juice, lemon peel and salt in a large bowl until sugar dissolves. Whisk in buttermilk.

2. Divide mixture among ice pop molds. Cover and freeze until firm (at least 4 hours).

Recipe #63:
Lemon Meringues

Lemon meringue is an old dessert favorite, and one that is sure to earn you some street cred with your friends when you have them over for dinner. These gorgeous little meringues are perfect for a small bite so you don't go overboard, but they pack a seriously delicious punch!

Ingredients:

- 2 large egg whites, at room temperature
- Pinch salt
- 2/3 cup sugar, sifted
- 1 tsp finely grated lemon zest
- 1/4 tsp vanilla extract
- Lemon sorbet (optional)

Equipment:

- Baking sheets
- Parchment paper
- Piping bag (optional)

Instructions:

1. Preheat oven to 250°F. The meringues must bake slowly to get the right consistency!

2. Cover two baking sheets with parchment paper.

3. Beat egg whites with salt until soft peaks form. Add sugar very slowly, beating well between additions, until egg whites are stiff but not dry. Fold in lemon zest and vanilla.

4. Drop teaspoonfuls onto the baking sheets or pipe small amounts with a pastry bag, fitted with a 1/2-inch star tip. Bake until dry but not brown, about 40 to 45 minutes. Cool 2 to 3 minutes before removing from the baking sheets.

5. Serve with lemon sorbet if desired!

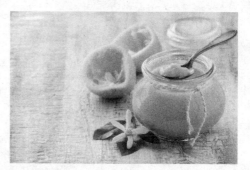

Recipe #64:
Lemon Curd with Honey

Lemon curd is an amazingly delicious topping to have in the fridge. It can be used on a wide range of things, from adding to your morning bowl of oatmeal for a tart infusion, to making decadent desserts and healthy baked goods that are a cut above the rest. Your only problem will be trying to resist eating it every time you open the fridge door!

Ingredients:

- 3 large free-range eggs
- 1/4 cup raw honey
- Zest of 2 organic lemons
- 1/4 cup coconut oil or unsalted butter (use expeller pressed/refined coconut oil if you do not want any coconut flavor)
- 1/3 cup plus 1 tbsp freshly squeezed lemon juice

Equipment:

- Saucepan
- Strainer or food mill
- Glass jar for storage

Instructions:

1. Mix eggs, honey and zest in a saucepan. Heat over medium-low heat and stir well.

2. Add coconut oil or butter and continue to stir constantly. Once it is melted, add the lemon juice.

3. Continue to cook over medium-low heat with constant stirring. The mixture will thicken to about the consistency of jam after 5 to 10 minutes. Be careful not to let the eggs scramble.

4. Place a strainer over your storage jar and pour the lemon curd in. Store in the refrigerator.

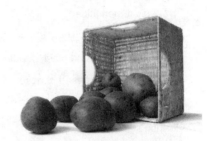

Recipe #65:
Lemon Potato Salad Bites

Guilt-free delicious snacks or appetizers are particularly hard to come by, but these tasty lemony bites deliver on that promise. They're packed with nutritious ingredients like avocado oil and lemon juice, and have a delicious rich buttery undertone that'll have you going back for more. Try to use organic ingredients where possible, and use grass-fed butter to take the health-giving powers of this dish to a whole new level.

Ingredients:

- 12 small red potatoes, halved (about 1 1/4 pounds)
- 2 tsp avocado oil
- 1/2 cup organic sour cream
- 2 tbsp minced fresh green onions
- 2 tbsp butter, melted
- 2 tbsp finely chopped drained capers

- 1 1/2 tsp lemon juice
- 1/2 tsp kosher salt
- 1/2 tsp freshly ground black pepper
- 2 tbsp grated Parmesan cheese

Equipment:

- Baking sheet
- Parchment paper

Instructions:

1. Preheat oven to 450°F.

2. Coat the potatoes lightly with avocado oil and arrange on a papered baking sheet, cut sides down. Bake for 20 to 30 minutes, then leave to cool.

3. Turn broiler to high.

4. Using a small knife, scoop out most of the insides of the potatoes leaving a thin shell.

5. In a mixing bowl, combine the scooped-out potato with sour cream, 1 tablespoon of green onions, butter, capers, lemon juice, salt and pepper. Mix well.

6. Fill the potato shells with the filling you've just made. Sprinkle with Parmesan and the remaining green onions.

7. Broil for 2 minutes or until cheese appears lightly toasted. Serve with extra sour cream.

Recipe #66:
Lemon Protein Bars

If you don't want to be caught hungry when you're out on the go and be forced to eat some nasty vending machine snack or sugary café-baked good, these lemon protein bars are just the things you need. They make a perfect transportable snack that will fill you up and give you energy. Best of all, they won't undermine your otherwise impeccable (we hope!) diet. Make a batch of these at the start of the week and always have one with you for when those mid-afternoon munchies hit.

Ingredients:

- 1 cup almond flour
- 2 scoops good quality whey protein (or hemp protein)
- 1/4 tsp salt
- 1/2 tsp baking soda
- Juice of 1 lemon
- 4 free-range eggs
- 1/2 cup raw honey
- 8 oz applesauce
- 1/2 tsp vanilla extract
- 4 oz water

Equipment:

- Glass baking dish

Instructions:

1. Grease the baking dish with coconut oil and preheat the oven to 350°F.

2. In a bowl, start with eggs, applesauce, honey, vanilla, water and lemon juice. Mix well.

3. Add flour, salt, baking soda and protein powder. Mix well until smooth.

4. Pour the mixture into greased baking dish, and bake about 20 minutes, or until the mixture is set and the top is slightly golden.

5. Slice into easy-to-transport bars and wrap so you can easily throw them in your purse or lunch bag.

Recipe #67: Lemon Cocktail

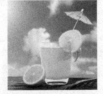

Let's face it: the fun hasn't really started until someone opens a bottle of vodka. No, we're not talking about just slugging back vodka straight from the bottle — that would be a little excessive! But a delicious lemony cocktail? Don't mind if we do, thanks. The focal point of this cocktail is, of course, some nice fresh lemon, which adds an amazing tartness that offsets the vodka nicely. It's somewhat addictive, so try not to get too carried away!

Ingredients:

- 2 cups freezer-chilled vodka

- 1/2 cup freshly squeezed lemon juice

- 1 lemon, thinly sliced

- 1/2 cup superfine sugar

Equipment:

- Cocktail shaker

Instructions:

1. Pour the vodka, lemon juice and sugar into a cocktail shaker with some crushed ice. Shake for around 30 seconds.

2. Pour the mixture into martini glasses and garnish with 1 slice of lemon per glass. Enjoy!

Wow, that's a lot of lemons! Lemons are so diverse and compliment so many different foods. They make a great addition to the kitchen, to the cleaning cupboard, and to your beauty regime! We hope you enjoy experimenting with all of the awesome benefits of lemons!

This page intentionally left blank.